...ni-Guide

ɔɪ **Misuse**

About the authors

Ken Barrie is a senior lecturer in Alcohol and Drug Studies in the School of Social Sciences at the University of the West of Scotland, where he has worked for 30 years. He is the programme leader for the MSc/Postgraduate Programme in Alcohol and Drug Studies. His main interests are treatment interventions and services for problem drinkers and drug users as well as public policy interventions as means of reducing harm. He has conducted commissioned research on substance use issues and service design for public bodies. He is currently investigating the links between poverty and problem substance use. His most recent book is *Alcohol* (2012). He is a member of the Society for the Study of Addiction.

Angela Scriven is Reader in Health Promotion at Brunel University in London, UK. She has been teaching and researching in the field of health promotion for more than 30 years and has published widely, including authoring, editing or co-editing the following books: *Health Promotion Alliances: Theory and Practice* (1998), *Health Promotion: Professional Perspectives* (1996, 2001), *Promoting Health: Global Perspectives* (2005), *Health Promoting Practice: The Contribution of Nurses and Allied Health Professionals* (2005), *Public Health: Social Context and Action* (2007), *Promoting Health: A Practical Guide* (2010), *Health Promotion for Health Practitioners* (2010), and *Health Promotion Settings: Principles and Practice*. Her research centres on the relationship between health promotion policy and practice within specific contexts. She is a member of the International Union of Health Promotion and Education (IUHPE), is President Elect of the Institute of Health Promotion and Education (IHPE), and is a Fellow of the Royal Society for Public Health (RSPH).

For Elsevier
Content Strategist: *Mairi McCubbin*
Content Development Specialist: *Barbara Simmons*
Project Manager: *Umarani Natarajan*
Designer/Design Direction: *Miles Hitchen*

Public Health Mini-Guide
Alcohol Misuse

Ken Barrie
Senior Lecturer in Alcohol and Drug Studies, School of Social Sciences,
University of the West of Scotland, Paisley, Scotland

Angela Scriven
Reader in Health Promotion, Brunel University, London, UK

Series editor:
Angela Scriven

CHURCHILL
LIVINGSTONE

ELSEVIER

Edinburgh London New York Oxford Philadelphia St Louis Sydney Toronto 2014

CHURCHILL
LIVINGSTONE
ELSEVIER

ISBN 9780702046384
Reprinted 2015

British Library Cataloguing in Publication Data
A catalogue record for this book is available from the British Library

Library of Congress Cataloging in Publication Data
A catalog record for this book is available from the Library of Congress

Notices

Knowledge and best practice in this field are constantly changing. As new research and experience broaden our understanding, changes in research methods, professional practices, or medical treatment may become necessary.

Practitioners and researchers must always rely on their own experience and knowledge in evaluating and using any information, methods, compounds, or experiments described herein. In using such information or methods they should be mindful of their own safety and the safety of others, including parties for whom they have a professional responsibility.

With respect to any drug or pharmaceutical products identified, readers are advised to check the most current information provided (i) on procedures featured or (ii) by the manufacturer of each product to be administered, to verify the recommended dose or formula, the method and duration of administration, and contraindications. It is the responsibility of practitioners, relying on their own experience and knowledge of their patients, to make diagnoses, to determine dosages and the best treatment for each individual patient, and to take all appropriate safety precautions.

To the fullest extent of the law, neither the Publisher nor the authors, contributors, or editors, assume any liability for any injury and/or damage to persons or property as a matter of products liability, negligence or otherwise, or from any use or operation of any methods, products, instructions, or ideas contained in the material herein.

ELSEVIER your source for books, journals and multimedia in the health sciences
www.elsevierhealth.com

 Working together to grow libraries in developing countries

www.elsevier.com • www.bookaid.org

The Publisher's policy is to use **paper manufactured from sustainable forests**

Printed in China

For Nancy

Contents

Titles in the Public Health Mini-Guide *series*:

Obesity
Nick Townsend, Angela Scriven
ISBN 9780702046346

Alcohol Misuse
Ken Barrie, Angela Scriven
ISBN 9780702046384

Diabetes (forthcoming)
Josie Evans, Angela Scriven
ISBN 9780702046377

Series preface

In the Foreword to its strategy for public health in England, the *Healthy Lives, Healthy People* White Paper (The Stationery Office, 2010), the UK government highlighted some of the public health challenges facing those working to improve public health: 'Britain is now the most obese nation in Europe. We have among the worst rates of sexually transmitted infections recorded, a relatively large population of problem drug users and rising levels of harm from alcohol. Smoking alone claims over 80,000 lives in every year. Experts estimate that tackling poor mental health could reduce our overall disease burden by nearly a quarter. Health inequalities between rich and poor have been getting progressively worse'. The public health targets are clear, both in the White Paper and in *Our Health and Wellbeing Today* (Department of Health, 2010), which was published to accompany the White Paper. The targets include policies for mental health, tobacco control, obesity, sexual health, and overall health.

The proposals and priorities identified in the White Paper apply to England, but they are of equal concern in the Devolved Administrations and globally, as evidenced in World Health Organization (WHO) reports (www.who.int/whr/en/index.html). The *Public Health Mini-Guides* series covers some of the key health targets identified by the UK government and WHO. The *Mini-Guides* highlight, in a concise, easily accessible manner, what the problems are and the range of potential solutions available to those professionals who have a responsibility to promote health.

What the *Public Health Mini-Guides* provide

The *Mini-Guides* are written to provide up-to-date, evidence-based information in a convenient pocket-sized format on a range of current key public health topics. They support the work of health and social care practitioners and students on courses related to public health and health promotion. Each volume provides an objective and balanced introduction to an overview of the epidemiological, scientific, and other factors relating to public health. The *Mini-Guides* are structured to provide easy access to information. The first chapters cover background information needed to quickly understand the issue, including epidemiology, demography, and physiology. The later chapters explore examples of public health action to address the issue, covering health promotion interventions and legislative and other measures. The *Mini-Guides* are designed to be essential reference texts for students, practitioners, and researchers who have a professional interest in public health and health promotion.

Uxbridge   Angela Scriven

References

Department of Health, 2010. Our Health and Wellbeing Today. Department of Health, London.
The Stationery Office, 2010. Healthy Lives, Healthy People. White Paper.

Preface

Alcohol is the UK's favourite psychoactive substance, and the production, sale and consumption of alcoholic beverages is a major element of the UK economy. Alcohol use is central to most ethnic, social, and cultural groups in the UK. The impact of alcohol on health, morbidity and mortality and the social fabric (family, crime and employment) is significant both at an individual and a population level. As alcohol has become cheaper and more available, associated problems have increased. Globally, a large proportion of disease is attributed to alcohol consumption, and alcohol places a burden not only on the individual but also on society as a whole. It is a major public health challenge on a global scale.

This mini guide presents key themes relating to this challenge, including the means of measuring alcohol use and related problems, the most recent prevalence and trends, the health and social consequences, and causes of alcohol misuse, along with approaches to reduce alcohol problems at an individual and a population level.

Chapter 1 covers the prevalence of alcohol use and drinking patterns in terms of regional, ethnic, social, and gender differences in the UK. The effects of alcohol, including cultural influences on conduct, are outlined. Definitions of risk and safer drinking limits are considered. Chapter 2 explores the health and social consequences of drinking. The role of alcohol in offending is evaluated. Health inequality and deprivation are considered as drivers of alcohol-related problems. Chapter 3 examines recovery from alcohol dependence, with and without treatment interventions. Evidence-based psychosocial and pharmacological interventions are described, as is the importance of the therapeutic alliance.

Chapter 4 focuses on two important social networks: the family and the workplace. The impact on both is considered, and the potential for both the family and workplace to influence recovery and prevention is explored. Chapter 5 emphasizes three important public health themes: the price of alcohol (including minimum unit pricing), control of the drinking environment, and alcohol education. Opposition to controls on alcohol by vested interests is appraised. Chapter 6 considers the evidence for reducing alcohol consumption and related problems among hazardous and harmful drinkers through contact with nonalcohol specialist services using screening techniques and alcohol brief interventions. Obstacles to progress, particularly in relation to professional education and attitudes, are explored.

Each chapter covers important content on these themes and includes suggestions where readers can find more information through links to Web pages, resources, and further reading. Understanding is facilitated through case studies, boxed examples, Thinking Points, and an end-of-chapter set of Summary Points.

1   Alcohol consumption

Europe has the largest consumption of alcohol in the world, with heavy episodic drinking widespread across all ages and all countries (WHO Europe, 2010). The measurement of alcohol consumption patterns in the UK is derived from sales data and drinking survey responses linked to recommended limits. These measurements show that consumption levels and drinking patterns vary across age, gender, ethnicity and social background, and there are recognised regional, national and international differences (Barrie, 2012). Alcohol is the UK's favourite and most commonly used psychoactive drug. The use of alcohol is embedded in UK culture, and alcohol is used for a number of purposes, including to celebrate and to commiserate. As alcohol has become cheaper and more available, more opportunities to drink it have arisen. Some sections of the drinking population in the UK are interested in the intoxicating effects achieved by binge drinking, but everyone who consumes alcohol does it because of the short-term effects (Marks, 2012).

Short-term effects of alcohol consumption

Alcohol is consumed for short-term benefits, usually the effect of the alcohol itself as well as the meaning that drinking alcohol conveys in a particular social setting or drinking culture (Banks, 2003). Observable changes in behaviour are a result of the depressant effect of alcohol on the central nervous system.

Observable behavioural, cognitive and physical changes resulting from alcohol consumption are (Paton, 2005):
- Slurring or thickening of speech
- Unsteady gait and staggering
- Deterioration of hand–eye coordination and reaction time
- Cognition change, including a deterioration in judgement
- Unconsciousness

These changes may be associated with the pleasure derived from drinking alcohol, as well as the negative consequences associated with intoxication, including accidents and social disorder. The effects of alcohol vary in different individuals. There is no guarantee that breath or blood alcohol measures will be similar in two individuals who have consumed the same amount of alcohol, even if they are of the same sex, age and weight. Similarly, three males with an identical blood or breath alcohol measure may have achieved this measure or level of intoxication by drinking different amounts. A breath alcohol measure of 35 µg per 100 ml breath (the current legal driving limit in the UK) may be achieved in the following examples:

Male 1 drinks about 4 or 5 units of alcohol (two pints of 5% by volume beer) in an hour.

Male 2 drinks a larger amount of alcohol over a longer period of time.

Male 3 drinks heavily the previous evening and takes the breath alcohol measure test at eight o'clock in the morning.

Irrespective of the consumption pattern, all three men would be breaking the law if they drove a car.

Women have a higher fat-to-water ratio in their bodies than men. As alcohol is not fat soluble, women will achieve a higher alcohol concentration (measured by blood or breath) when consuming amounts of alcohol equivalent to men, so women will become more intoxicated. On average, alcohol is eliminated from the body at a rate of about 1 unit per hour. Consequently, it will take longer to sober up if a larger quantity of alcohol is consumed. Despite biological measures of intoxication, individuals' descriptions of being intoxicated or drunk are very idiosyncratic (see https://www.drinkaware.co.uk/ for more information on alcohol consumption and intoxication).

Over time, individuals tend to become more tolerant of alcohol, that is, they are able to consume greater amounts of alcohol without necessarily appearing more intoxicated. So, while a novice 15-year-old drinker might feel drunk after consuming a litre of strong cider, a 22-year-old who consumes alcohol regularly would not be so affected and would need to consume significantly more to achieve the same effect. Tolerance may be similar to memory, whereby a similar tolerance level is retained or remembered after a period of reduced drinking or abstinence (Tiffany, 1990).

Drinking alcohol is known to cause a wide range of behaviours; exuberance and extraversion, talkativeness, wit and humour, sadness, amorousness, sexual arousal, aggression and violence. On an individual basis, some people (Heath, 2000) attribute certain behaviours to specific beverages, such as gin makes people sad and whisky makes people aggressive. However, it is not pharmacologically possible for one depressant (alcohol) to produce this range of behaviours. To explain alcohol-related behaviour, one must consider aspects of the individual and the social setting or culture in addition to pharmacology. Diverse cultures use alcohol for a variety of purposes without necessarily resulting in the negative outcomes noted in some drinking populations, such as aggression and violence (Young et al., 2007). Additionally, balanced placebo experiments suggest that individuals behave in a manner consistent with their belief about how much alcohol they have consumed, even when they have consumed a placebo (an alcohol-free drink). These experiments support the role of expectancy and sociocultural influences on drinkers' behaviour (Rohsenow and Marlatt, 1981).

Davies and Walsh (1983) established the guiding principle for a public health perspective on alcohol, which is that alcohol problems are the interaction of alcohol (agent), drinkers (host) and the physical and social environments.

Drinking culture

Most societies consist of more than one drinking culture, reflecting differences in geography, ethnicity, social class and age. Certain beverages and patterns of drinking may be more associated with certain sub-cultures, such as youth culture. While drinking cultures do change over time, they also reflect a history of a particular social or ethnic group. Similarly, a drinking culture is a means of passing on a set of rules and beliefs about alcohol from one generation to the next, so that young people are

socialised into the drinking culture as they are into many other aspects of adult life (Valentine et al., 2010).

Informal influences

Drinking cultures consist of a variety of values and attitudes about drinking, which provide a set of rules that are informally passed on, commonly by families and other social networks. In a culture where alcohol is highly acceptable, children are socialised into the drinking culture when they are quite young, long before they actually consume alcohol. At a young age, children have a concept of alcohol; at 4 years old, they can distinguish between "alcohol" bottles and other drink bottles, and at 6 years old, on seeing a video of a person staggering, children will conclude that the person is drunk, rather than ill. Young people in the UK are commonly introduced to alcohol by family members and over time observe and learn behavioural norms associated with consumption and conduct under the influence. This implies that aggression or violence is not simply a function of the amount of alcohol consumed but the extent to which such behaviour is culturally sanctioned: not everyone becomes aggressive under the influence of even quite large quantities of alcohol. Beyond family influence, religious affiliation and peer groups, the marketing of alcohol may create and support certain beliefs about the acceptability of alcohol and patterns of drinking. While informal influences may support alcohol consumption, they are also likely to offer guidelines about the time and place for drinking, limits of consumption and conduct under the influence (Percy, 2011).

A society with strong attachments to alcohol and intoxication will have a rich vocabulary on the subject of intoxication or drunkenness. BBC news reports that 'e-encyclopedia' has produced a glossary of 141 euphemisms for being drunk, suggested by the audience of a British Broadcasting Corporation (BBC) TV programme (http://news.bbc.co.uk/2/hi/uk_news/1883481.stm.). Suggestions were provided from across the UK, Ireland and further afield. A sample of these slang terms is shown in Box 1.1.

Most terms for drunkenness imply quite marked intoxication and therefore do not distinguish between differing degrees of drunkenness. This indicates the importance of drinking and intoxication in UK culture. Some terms for drunkenness are very old, others less so. There tends to be significant regional variation, though some terms are known and in current use nationally.

Formal influences

Alcohol is legal and subject to an array of regulations restricting access and availability (such as laws restricting hours of sale and age of drinkers). The price of alcohol is influenced by government-set taxation, and, in some instances, the price of alcohol may be influenced by public health interests. At a formal level, conduct under the influence or

---

Box 1.1 Slang terms used to describe being drunk

Banjaxed, Battered, Befuggered, Bernard Langered, Bladdered, Blasted, Blathered, Bleezin, Blitzed, Blootered, Blottoed, Brahms & Liszt, Buckled, Burlin,
Cabbaged, Chevy Chased, Clobbered, Decimated, Dot Cottoned, Druck-steaming, Drunk as a Lord, Drunk as a skunk, Etched,
Fecked, Four to the floor, Gatted, Goosed, Got my beer goggles on, Guttered, Hammered, Howling,
Inebriated, Intoxicated, Jahalered, Jaiked up, Jolly, Kaned,
Lagged up, Lamped, Langered, Laroped, Lashed, Leathered, Legless,
Mad wey it, Mandoo-ed, Mangled, Manky, Mashed, Meff'd, Merl Haggard, Merry, Ming-ho, Minging, Moired, Monged,
Off me trolley, Out of it, Out yer tree,
Rat-legged, Rubbered, Ruined,
Pickled, Pie-eyed, Pished, Plastered, Poleaxed, Pollatic,
Schindlers, Screwed, Scuttered, Slaughtered, Sloshed, Smashed, Snobbled, Sozzled, Spangled, Spannered, Spiffed, Spongelled, Squiffy, Steamin, Steampigged, Stocious, Stonkin,
Tanked, Tashered, Tipsy, Trashed, Trollied, Wasted, Wellied, With the fairies, Wrecked, Zombied.

Source: http://news.bbc.co.uk/1/hi/uk/1883481.stm (accessed 05/08/2013)

drunkenness is punished by the criminal justice system, which acknowledges alcohol offences, including drunk driving and other offences where alcohol may play a part. Alcohol production is a major economic activity, and alcohol is widely advertised in the UK, resulting in widespread images designed to encourage drinking. The existence of prevention policies and the provision of services for those suffering from alcohol-related consequences, including dependence on alcohol, are also part of drinking culture.

Different religions provide direction about alcohol, ranging from prohibition to appropriate use in given circumstances, including ceremonial use. Religious affiliation and increased religious observance tend to ameliorate problem drinking because religions offer guidance on drinking in moderation and on abstinence (Neighbors et al., 2013).

There is an interplay between elements of culture and formal influences on alcohol consumption. Changes in alcohol use by British young adults will therefore reflect not only the ebbs and flows of fashion and taste but also government, local authority and alcohol beverage industry policy (Measham, 2004).

Alcohol content

From brewing and distillation processes, a wide range of alcoholic beverages are produced, which range in strength from low-alcohol beers at 1% alcohol by volume (ABV) to cask strength spirits at around 60% ABV, with many beverages in between. Irrespective of the production method or type of beverage, a unit of alcohol is 10 g of pure alcohol (ethanol). Table 1.1 outlines the unit

Table 1.1 Units of alcohol and ABV in common beverages and bottle size

BEVERAGE	UNIT EQUIVALENT	ABV (%)	BOTTLE/ UNITS	VARIATIONS IN ABV
Beer	Half pint (235 ml) of "ordinary strength" beer	3.5–4	50 cl/2–3	5–7% ABV is common
Cider	Half pint (235 ml) of "ordinary strength" cider	3.5–4	2 l/8–16	6–8% ABV is common
Table wine	A small glass of table wine (125 ml)	9–10	70 cl/6–9	12–13% ABV is common
Fortified wine	35 ml measure	15–20	70 cl/ 11–14	Some contain caffeine
Spirits	25 ml measure	40	70 cl/28	Often sold in 35 ml measures

Source: http://www.healthscotland.com/uploads/documents/9344-Alcofacts2009.pdf (accessed 13/09/2013).

equivalent in relation to ABV of alcoholic beverages commonly sold in the UK, the number of units commonly found in a bottle, and variations commonly found in ABV in the same beverage, depending on strength.

Measuring alcohol consumption on the basis of units is complicated by the extent to which many beverages (beer, cider, wine) are available in higher ABV than the unit equivalent. Table wines are commonly 12–13% ABV, and beers and ciders are commonly available at 6% and 8% ABV, respectively. Therefore, it is possible for some beverages, such as table wine, to contain up to 50% more ABV. Some fortified wines, sometimes labelled as tonic wines, contain caffeine; however, while this may change the effect of the beverage, it does not alter the ABV. Spirits are sold in licensed premises in 25 ml

measures (1 unit); however, in Scotland 35 ml measures are common (40% greater alcohol content than the standard unit used in UK drinking surveys).

Recommended guidelines

UK government and health authorities have created recommended alcohol consumption levels for men and women in an attempt to inform the public, influence alcohol consumption and reduce levels of consumption that have the potential to result in harm (hazardous drinking) or that do cause harm (harmful drinking) (Department of Health, 1995). Given the details outlined in Table 1.2, it is not surprising to find that accurate recollection of the guidelines on alcohol consumption is limited.

Table 1.2 Drinking guidelines

QUANTITY	MEN	WOMEN
Daily		
Recommended/safe daily[a]	3–4 units maximum	2–3 units maximum
Pregnancy		0 units daily: 1–2 maximum
Binge: daily amounts	More than 8 units	More than 6 units
Weekly		
Recommended/safe weekly	21 units maximum	14 units maximum
Hazardous	22 + units per week	15 + units per week
Harmful	50 + units per week	36 + units per week

[a]Recommended or safer consumption guidelines suggest that people should refrain from drinking 2 days per week.
Source: http://www.healthscotland.com/uploads/documents/9344-Alcofacts2009.pdf (accessed 13/09/2013).

Guidelines in the UK recommend that men and women drink no more than 21 and 14 units of alcohol per week, respectively. On a daily basis, this amounts to 3–4 units per day for men and 2–3 units per day for women, with two alcohol-free days per week. There are different views on drinking during pregnancy, ranging from abstention to a maximum of 1–2 units of alcohol per day, once or twice a week (Burns et al., 2010). However, all UK chief medical officers advise that women who are pregnant or trying to conceive should avoid alcohol (Scottish Government, 2008). The Commons Select Committee Report (2012) on Alcohol Guidelines gives an overview of the evidence on which the alcohol advice that is publicised in the UK is based.

Levels and patterns of consumption

Abstinence

In 2009, 85% of adults were alcohol consumers, ranging from light/occasional drinking to harmful drinking, and 12% of men and 18% of women were abstainers. About 30% of men and 40% of women in both England and Scotland had not had an alcoholic drink in the previous week (Bromley and Shelton, 2010). Levels of abstinence were at their greatest among women over 65 years old. Only 10% of men 25–64 years old were abstainers. Some abstainers reported that they had always been a non-drinker

(57%), and 43% of abstainers reported that they had given up drinking. Among those who had never drunk, almost half said they didn't like drinking, while more than a quarter stated religious reasons for abstaining. Of those who had given up drinking, more than half stated that they abstained for health reasons (ONS, 2011).

Hazardous drinking

Men who drink more than 21 units per week and women who drink more than 14 units of alcohol per week are considered to be drinking hazardously. This relates to the risk or potential for harm or negative consequences as a result of drinking, irrespective of whether these consequences actually occur. For example, a man who drinks 4 pints (8 units) of beer per day may not experience any problems; however, there are always short- and long-term risks (e.g. accidents and chronic health problems).

Hazardous drinking is not a diagnostic term and is defined by WHO (1994) as a pattern of substance use that increases the risk of harmful consequences to the user. In contrast to harmful use, hazardous use refers to patterns of use that are of public health significance despite the absence of any current disorder in the individual. Men and women who consume more than 4 and 3 units of alcohol per day, respectively, are considered hazardous drinkers based on the government's guidelines on limits for alcohol consumption.

Among men, 37% and, among women, 20% exceeded the recommended limits. Hazardous drinkers are commonly identified through health care screening programmes. They are likely to be offered alcohol brief interventions (see Chapter 6 for details on brief interventions).

Harmful drinking

Men who consume more than 50 units of alcohol per week, or 8 units of alcohol per day, and women more than 35 units per week, or 6 units per day, are considered harmful drinkers. They will often show clear signs of alcohol-related damage (WHO, 1993), and a significant proportion of harmful drinkers are likely to be moderately to severely dependent on alcohol (Raistrick et al., 2006). Among men, 20% drank harmfully, and among women, 13% drank harmfully. (Alcohol dependence will be discussed in greater detail in Chapters 2 and 4.) When broken down by age, heavy or harmful drinking was noted more commonly in younger men and women (ONS, 2011).

A significantly lower proportion of Scottish men drank within the recommended guidelines (up to 4 units per day) when compared to men in England. Furthermore, Scottish men were more likely to drink in excess of these limits. Average consumption on heavy drinking days was almost 50% higher among Scottish men when compared to English men (6.2 and 4.3 units, respectively).

A significantly lower proportion of women drank within the recommended guidelines (up to 3 units per day) in Scotland compared to England. Average consumption on heavy drinking days was in excess of 50% higher among Scottish women when compared to English women (3.5 and 2.2 units, respectively). Consumption among women in Scotland was on average in excess of the recommended limits (2–3 units). In Scotland and England 18% and 15% of women, respectively, drank harmfully (more than 6 units on the heaviest drinking day). In both England and Scotland, significant proportions of men and women drank hazardously and harmfully in the previous 7 days. Levels of both hazardous and harmful alcohol consumption were noted to be higher in Scotland (Bromley and Shelton, 2010).

Binge drinking

There is no commonly agreed upon definition of binge drinking (Marks and O'Connor, 2011), and this fact is reflected in public perceptions of the term. Binge drinking reflects a style of drinking common to UK drinking culture. Scotland's Plan for Action on Alcohol (Scottish Executive, 2002) defined binge drinking as drinking an excessive amount on any one occasion. Men who drink more than 8 units per day and women who drink more than 6 units per day are also considered to be at risk of binge drinking even if they don't exceed the weekly safe drinking limit. Men and women are likely to suffer alcohol-related consequences when they regularly drink more than 8 units and 6 units, respectively, on a heavy drinking day (ONS, 2011), and this measure has become the conventional definition of binge drinking in UK population surveys. The essence of binge drinking is a pattern of high consumption, especially in a relatively short period of time, which thereby maximises the intoxicating effects of alcohol. However, by merely paying attention to the amount consumed on a daily basis, the nature of binge drinking can go unnoticed.

For example, if a man consumes 10 units of alcohol starting at midday and consumes 1 unit per hour, his blood alcohol measure wouldn't likely be more than 20 mg alcohol per 100 ml of blood (the legal limit for drunk driving in the UK is 80 mg alcohol per 100 ml of blood or 35 mg of alcohol per 100 ml of breath). While a large amount of alcohol may be consumed on one drinking day, the pattern of consumption can hardly be describes as a "binge", given that a high blood alcohol level is never achieved and "drunken behaviour" may not be observed.

It may be that a more subjective measure, such as reporting "feeling drunk" or "feeling very drunk", is a better indicator of binge drinking than the amounts of alcohol consumed (SALSUS, 2008).

Many harmful drinkers are binge drinkers, as their drinking pattern consists of a regular high-volume drinking day; most harmful drinking could be described as a "binge", as distinct from a "risky single occasion" of drinking, where high consumption is irregular, for example, weekly (Gmel et al., 2011). The persistent high volume, serial binge drinking of the harmful drinker tends to result in chronic health and social consequences, whereas the risky single-occasion harmful drinker will more commonly experience problems associated with accidents and social disorder.

In a study of higher education students in Scotland, Marks and O'Connor (2011) interviewed over 300 students (mean age 23, range 16–58 years), of whom 80% were female; 65% of the sample fit the criteria for "binge" drinkers. This style of alcohol consumption, given the large proportion of the sample fitting the criteria, may be considered normal in the UK. When binge drinkers were compared with non-binge drinkers, no differences in ethnicity, social class, employment status or gender were found. However, binge drinkers were more likely to report drinking to be sociable, to conform, to forget worries and for excitement. They also reported higher levels of alcohol-related consequences, stress and depression as well as drinking at an earlier age. Interestingly, frequency of hangovers predicted symptoms of depression (Paljarva et al., 2009).

Binge drinking is associated with increased risk for injuries and some diseases (Rehm et al., 2010; Gmel et al., 2011). In a study comparing 10,000 male drinkers from France and Northern Ireland, followed up over a 10-year period, 9% of middle-aged Irish males were found to be binge drinkers, most commonly at weekends, compared to 0.5% in France. Around 75% of French men drank daily, but less alcohol per drinking session, compared to 12% of men from Northern Ireland. Binge drinkers had almost twice the risk of heart attack or death from heart disease compared with regular drinkers (Ruidavets et al., 2010). Clearly, binge drinking is not simply an activity associated with younger people; its widespread existence across the population suggests that it is culturally driven.

Alcohol expenditure and sales

In 2000, the expenditure in the UK for alcohol was £38.5 billion, rising to a peak of £44.4 billion in 2004 and falling subsequently to £37 billion in 2009, at constant 2006 prices. In 2000, in Scotland total sales were £3.64 billion, reflecting a 9% increase from 2005. From 2005 to 2009, on-trade sales increased by 1% while sales at off-trade establishments increased by 22%. Modest decreases in beer and spirit sales were outstripped by increases in sales of wine and cider. Between 2005 and 2009, total customer expenditures on all alcoholic beverages in the UK decreased less than 1%.

In Scotland between 2005 and 2009, the number of litres of pure alcohol sold remained fairly constant at 12 l per person over the age of 16 per year. During the same period, around 10 l of pure alcohol were sold per person per year in England and Wales. This indicates that alcohol sales in Scotland are 20% greater per person than in the rest of the UK. Across the UK, the downturn in on-trade sales and the upturn in off-trade sales are consistent with expenditure receipts for the same period. Similarly, in Scotland in 2005, there was a 40:60 ratio in on- versus off-trade sales, which shifted to a 30:70 ratio in 2009 (ISD, 2011).

Population surveys on alcohol behaviour

It is generally recognised that social surveys of drinking behaviour report lower levels of consumption than alcohol sales records. This may be due to individuals consciously or unconsciously underestimating their consumption, whether related to poor memory or a reluctance to divulge personal information. Impaired memory of the details of recent drinking sessions may lead to underestimation, particularly if a large amount of alcohol has been consumed. This underestimation may also be due to the difficulty in estimating home-poured drinks, which tend to be larger than those served in licensed premises. It is also possible that the heaviest alcohol consumers are not available or do not wish to participate in such surveys, leading to an insufficient or inaccurate sample being surveyed.

However, drinking surveys provide information that sales records cannot, namely, accounts of alcohol consumption in relation to volume and frequency of drinking. In addition, they provide information on associations between individual characteristics, such as age, gender, socio-economic background, region of residence and alcohol consumption, all of which may provide data needed to develop policy responses (ONS, 2011; ISD, 2011). The best picture of alcohol consumption is based on a variety of sources, including survey data and sales records.

Survey trends: mid 1990s to 2009 for UK adults
1998–2000

During the 1990s, the General Household Survey (GHS) reported a slight increase in alcohol consumption among men and a significantly greater increase among women. Following an increase between 1998 and 2000, a decline occurred in hazardous drinking among both men (29–23%) and women (17–12%). Surveys show little change between 1998 and 2003, a period of peak consumption, based on reported previous 7 days drinking or drinking in excess of recommended limits. A similar pattern emerged for harmful drinking among men and women, exceeding 8 and 6 units

on at least 1 day per week, respectively (Smith and Foxcroft, 2009).

2000–2006

Hazardous drinking in both men and women decreased between 2000 and 2006. This decrease was most noticeable in the 16–24 age group; among men, hazardous drinking decreased from 50% to 39%, and among women from 42% to 34%. The proportion of men drinking harmfully also decreased from 37% to 27% in this period (Smith and Foxcroft, 2009).

2006/2007–2009

More modest reductions were reported for 2007–2009, and this downward shift in consumption continued, which was reflected in alcohol sales data. There were reductions in the proportion of those reporting having had an alcoholic drink in the previous 7 days: 72–68% of men and 57–54% of women. Hazardous drinking among men decreased from 41% to 37% and from 34% to 29% among women. Harmful drinking decreased from 23% to 20% (men) and 15% to 13% (women) (Smith and Foxcroft, 2009).

From consumption levels which were at their highest at the turn of the century, there is a downward trend in consumption since around 2005 or 2006, which is confirmed by surveys and sales data. This may be partly a result of the current economic downturn.

> **! Thinking Point**
>
> What reasons can be attributed to the downward trend in alcohol consumption since 2005 or 2006?

National and regional differences in alcohol consumption

Table 1.3 shows the 2009 average reported weekly alcohol consumption of men and women in Wales, Scotland and England, with further detail from English regions. There were no significant differences in average weekly alcohol consumption among the countries of the UK. In England, the highest average weekly consumption was in the North East (14.4 units) and the lowest was in London and the West Midlands (both 9.3 units).

In 2009, 69% of men and 55% of women in England consumed alcohol in the previous week compared to 58% and 48%, respectively, in Scotland. Men in Wales and England were more likely than men in Scotland to have an alcoholic

Table 1.3 Average weekly adult alcohol consumption (in units) by gender, country and English region

COUNTRY/REGION	AVERAGE WEEKLY CONSUMPTION		
	Men	Women	Total
Wales	16.7	8.6	12.4
Scotland	15.0	7.8	11.2
England	16.4	8.0	11.9
English regions			
Northeast	21.0	9.4	14.4
Northwest	17.3	9.0	13.1
Yorkshire and Humber	17.7	9.8	13.6
East Midlands	16.3	7.8	11.9
West Midlands	14.0	6.9	10.2
East of England	15.8	7.8	11.6
London	13.4	6.0	9.3
South East	17.1	8.4	12.5
South West	17.6	7.9	12.2
UK	16.3	8.0	11.9

Source: Office of National Statistics (ONS), 2011.

drink on at least 5 days out of the previous 7 (17% and 19%, respectively, compared with 12%). The North East, North West and the Yorkshire and Humber region had the highest proportions of adults drinking more than 4/3 units (40%, 39% and 41%, respectively). These regions also had the highest levels of heavy drinking, which made them the highest-consuming regions in the UK.

Regional variations are more marked than national distinctions. On the basis of reported average weekly alcohol consumption, Scotland does not stand out, consuming less than Wales and all English regions with the exceptions of London and the West Midlands. However this is contradicted by sales records that show 20% higher per capita alcohol sales and consumption levels in Scotland compared to England (Bromley and Shelton, 2010; ISD, 2011).

Social and cultural influences on alcohol consumption

Drinking of children and young people

Surveys about drinking among young people (under the age of 16) are usually conducted using school students. More than half of Scottish 13 year olds and less than 40% of Scottish 15 year olds and 48% of 11–15 year olds in England who reported that they had ever had a drink indicated that they had never actually bought alcohol. Obtaining, or purchasing, alcohol from friends and relatives appears to be the most consistent and increasing source of alcohol for underage drinkers, as the percentage of those reporting purchase directly from off-licence and on-licence premises has significantly decreased since the early 1990s. While this trend may reflect increased vigilance about underage drinking on the part of licence holders (both on- and off-licence), it also reflects the general shift toward purchasing from off-licence premises (including supermarkets) at lower prices as well as a permissive attitude toward adults giving alcohol to younger people. Alcohol advertising and sponsorship also contributes to a positive attitude toward alcohol among younger people, which is predictive of subsequent drinking (Babor et al., 2003).

Among 13 and 15 year olds in Scotland, 52% and 82%, respectively, indicated that they had consumed an alcoholic drink. Similar proportions reported having been "really drunk" at least once. Approximately 50% of English young people who drank in the previous 4 weeks reported feeling drunk (58% of girls and 49% of boys). Around 40% of 13 year olds and 55% of 15 year olds in Scotland reported at least one from a list of negative consequences associated with alcohol intoxication, the most common being "having an argument" and "vomiting". Self-reported drunkenness appears to be more common among Scottish young people. The experience of drunkenness increases with age, and heavier drinking among young people is commonly associated with use of tobacco and other drugs (SALSUS, 2008).

In Scotland between 2006 and 2008, there was a decrease from 14% to 11% of 13 year olds and from 36% to 31% of 15 year olds who reported consuming alcohol in the previous week. In the same period in England there was a decrease in 11–15 year olds who reported drinking alcohol in the previous week from 26% in 2006 to 18% in 2008 (NHSIC, 2010). While reported drinking in this age group is similar to that recorded in 1990, peaks of 20% and 47% (13 and 15 year olds, respectively) were recorded in 1996, peaking again in 2002 at 23% and 46% for 13 and 15 year olds, respectively (SALSUS, 2008; ISD, 2011). The changes in reported drinking in young people, in both countries, mirrored the reported consumption of the general adult population during the same period.

Socio-economic class

The Department of Health (1998), in an independent inquiry on health inequalities, noted a clear relationship between socio-economic class and morbidity and mortality. Death rates were noted to be significantly higher among unskilled men than those from professional households. Over a lengthy period, GHS (ONS, 2011) has shown little difference in the weekly consumption of alcohol between manual and non-manual households. Any difference identified tended to be in non-manual households, where higher consumption was associated with greater disposable income. A ministerial task force on health inequalities reached similar conclusions, with a strong emphasis on the role of alcohol, drugs and violence (Scottish Government, 2008a,b).

ONS (2011) reported that, in 2009 in the UK, average weekly alcohol consumption was highest, at 13.5 units, in the professional–managerial group, with 77% of men and 65% of women having an alcoholic drink in the previous 7 days and lowest at 10.7 units among those in manual households, where 59% of men and 44% of women had an alcoholic drink in the previous 7 days. This is a consistent finding for both men and women; however, the difference is greater when professional women are compared to women in manual households where their weekly consumption is 9.7 and 6.6 units per week, respectively.

Women in professional/managerial households were twice as likely to drink more than 3 units on any one day compared to women from manual households. They were also twice as likely to have drunk heavily on at least one occasion in the previous week. A similar, but smaller, distinction was apparent when comparing men from professional and manual households (Bromley and Shelton, 2010).

Thinking Point

What factors are likely to influence the
different alcohol consumption patterns
in professional/managerial households
and manual households?

Ethnicity

In the UK survey (NHSIC, 2010),
respondents of Pakistani or Bangladeshi
origin in the UK were unlikely to have
drunk in the previous week, 5% and 4%,
respectively, compared to 68% among
those who described themselves as "white
British". Such low levels of alcohol
consumption in a large ethnic community
could serve to reduce the average alcohol
consumption in particular geographical
areas. Ethnicity, on the basis of religious
affiliation, presents a contrasting
picture. Cochrane and Bal (1990)
investigated the alcohol consumption
of Sikh, Hindu, Muslim and white English

males in the West Midlands. Alcohol
consumption levels and patterns of
drinking among males from the different
ethnic groups were quite different, as were
the consequences of drinking. In Muslim
culture, where alcohol consumption is
expressly forbidden, those very few males
who did consume alcohol were very heavy
consumers and deviant from their cultural
and religious norms. The weekly
consumption of alcohol by the Sikh and
white English males was very similar.
However, when problems were
considered, the Sikhs reported family
problems in relation to their drinking,
while the white English males reported
much higher levels of "police trouble".
This reflects the regular drinking of Sikh
males compared to the binge-style
drinking of white English males and the
legal consequences that can ensue as well
as the different cultural influences
brought to bear on alcohol consumption
and related conduct.

Summary Points

- Per capita alcohol consumption has risen substantially in recent decades, reaching a
  peak in the middle of the first decade of the 21st century, followed by a modest
  decline.
- Current consumption, relative to preceding decades, is high.
- Consumption is sensitive to the price of alcohol and is in relation to overall
  consumer expenditure, so cheaper alcohol has resulted in increased consumption.
- Recent changes in the UK have contributed to the economic downturn from 2008
  onward, making alcohol relatively more expensive and, in turn, reducing
  consumption.
- Alcohol consumption is difficult to measure, given the range of strengths in which
  alcoholic beverages are available.

Continued

- There is a significant gap apparent between sales data and the responses given in surveys.
- Surveys present a broadly consistent picture of declining alcohol consumption in the early 21st century from 2006 to 2009.
- There has been a significant shift in sales from the on-trade licensed premises to off-trade or off-licence premises, including supermarkets, where price per unit of alcohol is significantly cheaper, altering drinking patterns and consequences as a result.
- Those with the highest income have the highest average consumption, have more occasions to drink, and are more likely to consume more alcohol than is recommended.
- Negative alcohol-related consequences, including health consequences, affect the less well off much more despite their more modest average consumption. See Chapter 2 for more details on health impacts.
- While there is a similarity in consumption levels between different ethnic groups, the reported social consequences of drinking are quite different. This reflects cultural differences in drinking patterns and in expectations related to conduct under the influence of alcohol.
- Drinking culture in the UK is diverse on the basis of age, gender, ethnicity and social background. "Binge" drinking is a normal part of drinking culture in the UK, though antisocial behaviour and health consequences associated with this pattern of drinking are major sources of public health concern.

Web pages and resources

http://www.nhs.uk/Livewell/alcohol/Pages/Bingedrinking.aspx
The NHS Choices webpage on binge drinking includes definitions and links to videos and tools on the safe use of alcohol.

http://www.drinkaware.co.uk/understand-your-drinking/is-your-drinking-a-problem/binge-drinking
Drinkaware is an independent, UK-wide charity. Their webpages provide a range of facts on binge drinking and alcohol consumption and a number of useful tools that can be personalised for individual monitoring of alcohol consumption patterns.

http://www.ons.gov.uk/ons/rel/lifestyles/drinking–adult-s-behaviour-and-knowledge/2009-report/index.html
The Office of National Statistics (ONS) data on alcohol behaviour in the UK is regularly updated and includes useful information on current trends.

http://www.euro.who.int/en/what-we-do/health-topics/disease-prevention/alcohol-use/facts-and-figures
The World Health Organisation Regional Office for Europe provides facts and figures on alcohol behaviour across the region.

http://www.jrf.org.uk/publications/drinking-in-the-uk
This link provides access to the report "Drinking in the UK: An exploration of trends", which reviews research and highlights trends in alcohol consumption over the last 20–30 years.

http://www.publications.parliament.uk/pa/cm201012/cmselect/cmsctech/1536/1536.pdf
This link takes you to the Commons Select Committee Report on Alcohol Guidelines. The report discusses in detail the evidence for the guidelines.

Further reading

Bécares, L., 2009. The ethnic density effect on alcohol use among ethnic minority people in the UK. J. Epidemiol. Commun. Health 65 (1), 20–25.

This study examines the hypothesis that ethnic minority people living in areas of high ethnic density will report less alcohol use relative to their counterparts, due to decreased experienced racism and increased sociocultural norms.

Craig, D.G., et al., 2011. A drunk and disorderly country: a nationwide cross-sectional survey of alcohol use and misuse in Great Britain. Frontline Gastroenterol. 3 (1), 57–63.
This chapter offers a critical overview of the current alcohol drinking patterns, behaviours and attitudes in Great Britain.

2 The health and legal consequences of problem drinking

The World Health Organisation European Region has the world's highest proportion of total estimated ill health and premature death caused by alcohol, and there is a very close relationship between a country's total per capita alcohol consumption and its prevalence of alcohol-related harm and alcohol dependence (WHO, 2010). Alcohol consumption in the UK and Scotland in particular seems high by European and global standards and has had an impact on the health, relationships, employment, and legal dimensions of people's lives (Box 2.1).

In the past decade, public concern has focused mainly on young people's binge drinking and the associated public disorder instead of alcohol's health impacts. In this chapter, we outline the relationship between alcohol and health, including alcohol dependence. Deprivation and health inequality are considered as contributory factors of both alcohol-related health consequences and offending behaviour.

Economic costs of problem drinking

Within the UK, it is difficult to estimate and compare the costs of alcohol-related health and social consequences. Devolved governments arrive at estimates based on the inclusion and exclusion of different criteria and in response to different public concerns. Furthermore, health, criminal justice, and social services are structured differently. Consequently, making comparisons among the nations of the UK is difficult. Nevertheless, the fact that costs have been attributed to alcohol-related consequences means that concerns about the magnitude of alcohol's impact and a drive for change based on economic expediency have emerged.

The Department of Health (DoH) estimates the costs to the National Health Service (NHS) in England and Wales at approximately £2.7 billion a year, and alcohol-related admissions account for

---

> **Box 2.1 Roizen's model: a useful shorthand for the harms that may be experienced through use of drugs**
>
> | | |
> |---|---|
> | Liver | Stands for all physical problems and also for psychological problems caused by drug use, such as depression, anxiety, and psychosis. |
> | Lover | Stands for problems with relationships, with family and/or friends. |
> | Livelihood | Refers to problems of employment, from being demoted to being sacked. Also includes problems with studies, financial problems, and other problems. |
> | Law | Refers to all the legal problems that may result from drug use. |
>
> *Source: http://toolboxes.flexiblelearning.net.au.*

7% of the total admissions to the NHS (NHSIC, 2010). The DoH (2012a,b) estimate the total annual costs of alcohol consumption in England and Wales, including losses to industry and commerce, to be about £21 billion. In Scotland, the 2007 alcohol-related costs of health care, including primary care, community-based care, and hospital care, were estimated to be about £269 million; most of these costs are attributable to alcohol-related hospital admissions. In Northern Ireland, in 2008–2009, it was estimated that the total costs of alcohol misuse could be as much as £900 million per year (DHSSPSNI, 2011). In Wales, the estimated cost to the NHS of alcohol-related chronic disease and acute incidents is between £70 and £85 million each year (Alcohol Concern, 2010a,b).

Social care costs associated with alcohol in Scotland were between £114 and £347 million (median £230 million) in 2007.

The majority of these costs are derived from social care relating to children and families; care homes; the Children's Hearing System and criminal justice social work, including probation services (Beale et al., 2009) (see Table 2.1).

Alcohol-related costs of £21 billion for England are modest compared to an estimate of £55 billion, which was provided by the National Social Marketing Centre:

- £21 billion cost to individuals and families/households
- £2.8 billion cost to public health services/care services
- £2.1 billion cost to other public services (e.g. criminal justice system costs, education costs, and social services costs)
- £7.3 billion cost to employers
- £21.9 billion in human costs (disability-adjusted life-years)

Source: www.publications.parliament.uk.

Table 2.1 The estimated health costs of problem drinking in the UK

NATION	HEALTH COST	JUSTICE COST	SOCIAL CARE	TOTAL
England and Wales[1]	£2.7 billion	£2.8 billion including social care		£21 billion[4]
Scotland[2]	£269 million	£727 million	£230 million	£1.23 billion
Northern Ireland[3]				£900 million

Source: [1]NHSIC (2010), [2]Beale et al. (2009), [3]DHSSPSNI (2011), [4]DoH (2012a,b).

Justice costs are explored further in the 'Alcohol and offending' section later in this chapter.

The relationships between alcohol and health

Alcohol contributes to 4% of the global burden of disease, which is the same level of death and disability globally as that associated with tobacco and hypertension (Room et al., 2005). The burden is higher still in those countries where both alcohol consumption and consequences are higher than the global average. This is most notable among the European nations, including the UK (Rehm et al., 2010).

Harm-free or safer drinking patterns

Drinking less than the government-recommended limits of 14 units of alcohol per week for women and 21 units per week for men is associated with reduced risk of alcohol-related health and social consequences and is a definition of harm-free or safer drinking

(see Chapter 1). However, reduced risk does not mean that there is no risk of alcohol-related consequences as, in some instances, any alcohol consumption is risky, such as when a person is driving or operating machinery. Low levels of alcohol consumption are associated with a reduction in the risk of cardiovascular heart disease in men over age 40 and women who are postmenopausal, where benefit can be gained by regularly drinking as little as one unit of alcohol per day. No additional health benefits result if more than two units per day are consumed. Studies of cancers indicate that there is no safe limit for alcohol consumption below which the risk of cancer is avoided though increased prevalence of cancers is associated with drinking in excess of recommended limits (Schutze et al., 2011). Therefore, a low level of consumption, which may be beneficial in preventing one particular disease, such as cardiovascular disease, will not necessarily prevent the occurrence of another, such as alcohol-related cancers. It is also widely acknowledged that any benefits accruing from very modest alcohol consumption can also be achieved by other means, such as exercise and diet.

Thinking Point

Do you think the number of recommended units of alcohol should be changed? If so, what would you change it to?

Heavy drinking patterns

While volume of alcohol consumed is associated with alcohol-related health problems, attention must also be paid to heavy drinking patterns. Modest consumption on a regular basis results in less harm to a population and individuals compared to heavy episodic drinking, that is, high levels of consumption on individual drinking occasions, commonly called *binge drinking* (see Chapter 1).

Binge drinking is associated with increased risk for all injuries and some diseases (Rehm et al., 2010; Gmel et al., 2011). In a study comparing 10,000 male drinkers in France and Northern Ireland over a 10-year period, 9% of middle-aged males in Belfast were found to be binge drinkers, most commonly at weekends, compared to 0.5% in France. Around 75% of French men drank daily, but consumed less per drinking session, compared to 12% of men from Northern Ireland. Binge drinkers had almost twice the risk of heart attack or death from heart disease compared to regular drinkers. Regular and moderate alcohol intake throughout the week, the typical

pattern in middle-aged men in France, is associated with a low risk of ischaemic heart disease, whereas the binge drinking pattern more prevalent in Belfast confers a higher risk (Ruidavets et al., 2010).

Members of the LGBT (lesbian, gay, bisexual, and transgender) community report binge drinking twice as often as the rest of the population (Keogh et al., 2009). In these groups, alcohol plays an important role in social and sexual contact just as it does in the heterosexual population. In particular, alcohol use by gay men is associated with an increased risk of engaging in risky or unprotected sex. Alcohol use facilitates engagement in sexual practices that are stigmatised when sober (Parsons et al., 2004). Consequently, there is an increased potential for passing on or contracting HIV (human immunodeficiency virus). Furthermore, such heavy drinking is associated with damage to the immune system and consequent seroconversion of HIV to AIDS (acquired immunodeficiency syndrome). Heavy consumption is also associated with poor adherence to antiretroviral medication and treatment outcomes (Rehm et al., 2010; HIV Scotland, 2012).

Alcohol and non-communicable diseases

Together with smoking, diet, and sedentary lifestyle, consumption of alcohol is considered to be among the most important risk factors for non-communicable diseases (NCDs) (Room and Rehm, 2011). Many acute and chronic diseases and injuries are affected by alcohol consumption and drinking patterns, with increased consumption associated with increased risk. Alcohol is causally related to more than 60 medical conditions (Room et al., 2005). In some cases, alcohol is wholly attributable as the cause of health conditions, which are listed in international disease classifications (ICD-10, WHO, 1992). Where alcohol is partly attributable, it is one of a number of causes. The proportionate contribution of alcohol may vary from one disease to another or vary for the same disease when women and men are compared. Diseases in which alcohol has a causal influence are outlined in Box 2.2.

Cancers

Researchers concluded that the burden of cancer attributed to both current and former drinkers in eight European countries, including the UK (Schutze et al., 2011), indicates that there was a causal link between alcohol consumption in 10% of cancers in males and 3% in

---

Box 2.2 Alcohol and its causal impact on major health consequences

Wholly attributable

tuberculosis
diabetes
alcoholic liver disease, including cirrhosis of the liver
alcohol use disorders
alcoholic polyneuropathy, myopathy, cardiomyopathy, gastritis and pancreatitis
alcohol-related degeneration of the nervous system (alcohol-related brain damage, including Wernicke–Korsakoff syndrome)
intentional and accidental poisoning by alcohol
epilepsy
unipolar depressive disorders
lower respiratory infections (pneumonia)
pre-term birth complications and FAS

Partly or proportionately attributable

cancers: mouth, nasopharynx, other pharynx and oropharynx, oesophageal cancer, colon and rectum cancer, liver cancer, breast cancer in women
hypertensive heart disease, ischaemic heart disease (IHD), ischaemic and haemorrhagic stroke, conduction disorders, and other dysrhythmias
injuries: road traffic accidents, fire injuries, assaults, accidents, and intentional self harm
psoriasis, epilepsy, spontaneous abortion

Source: Rehm et al. (2010), ISD (2011).

---

females in Europe, with a substantial proportion of cancers associated with consumption at levels greater than the recommended limits (Box 2.2). Alcohol is implicated in the prevalence of cancers in 8% of males and 3% of females in the UK. Compared to Europe, the prevalence in the UK is slightly lower for men but the same for women. The proportion of cancers attributable to alcohol increases markedly both in Europe and the UK when cancers with a wholly attributable causal relationship are considered: 32% and 5% in men and women, respectively.

Table 2.2 indicates that, with the exception of breast cancer, alcohol-attributed cancers are proportionately higher amongst men than women. The proportion of alcohol-attributed cancer incidence was highest in relation to cancers of the upper aerodigestive tract, where the proportion was slightly higher in the UK compared to Europe. This was followed by cancer of the liver, where the proportion was the same between men and lower for women in the UK compared to Europe.

> **! Thinking Point**
>
> Why do you think that alcohol-attributed cancers are proportionally higher in men than women?

Liver disease

The key drivers for the growth in the burden of and mortality from liver disease are all preventable: alcohol, obesity, hepatitis C, and hepatitis B (Effiong et al., 2012). In assessing end-of-life care needs, it was noted that deaths from liver disease in England have risen by 25% in less than a decade, from 9231 in 2001 to 11,575 in 2009. Liver disease deaths are more common among men than women (60%

Table 2.2 Proportion of cancer cases (in %) attributable to alcohol use in males and females age 15 or over: UK and Europe

CANCER	UK MEN (%)	UK WOMEN (%)	EUROPE MEN (%)	EUROPE WOMEN (%)
Total cancer	8	3	10	3
Alcohol-related cancers				
Upper aerodigestive tract[a]	45	30	44	25
Colorectum	14	5	17	4
Liver	33	13	33	18
Breast		5		5

[a]Upper aerodigestive tract cancers: oral cavity, pharynx, larynx, oesophagus.
Source: Schutze et al. (2011).

are men, 40% women). Younger age groups are disproportionately affected; 90% of people who die from liver disease are under 70 years old, and more than 10% of people who die from liver disease are in their forties. Alcoholic liver disease accounts for well over a third (37%) of liver disease deaths. Heavy or harmful drinking exacerbates liver disease later in life (Gibson et al., 2011). Among 1075 illicit drug users in England and Wales who entered treatment for drug problems, a significant proportion were drinking harmfully in addition to using illicit drugs (Gossop et al., 2003). Over the follow-up period of 5 years, significant reductions in illicit drug use and associated offending were noted, but there were no similar reductions in alcohol consumption. In a community drug service study in Scotland, O'Rawe (2007) reported harmful levels of alcohol consumption in a cohort of service users prescribed maintenance methadone, including about 20% who had been in contact with specialist alcohol services. Harmful drinking was more common among those who had been prescribed methadone for more than 5 years. Continued hazardous alcohol consumption may result in poor prognosis for hepatitis C and an increased demand for end-of-life care (Effiong et al., 2012).

Fertility and foetal alcohol effects

Alcohol affects fertility in women and is also associated with miscarriages. Modest alcohol consumption is recommended for women planning a pregnancy and very low or no alcohol consumption is recommended during pregnancy (Burns et al., 2010).

Alcohol is the most common substance associated with developmental abnormalities in the foetus, causing perhaps 10% of physical malformations, and is considered the most common cause of mental and behavioural problems in children (Abel and Sokol, 1986). Heavy consumption during pregnancy, especially during the first trimester, is associated with foetal alcohol effects (FAEs). Exact numbers are difficult to define in this spectrum of disorder, but it is estimated that FAEs occur in 3–5 per 1000 live births, and foetal alcohol syndrome (FAS) occurs in 1–2 per 1000 live births in the UK. FAS is a spectrum of disorders, varying in severity. FAEs represent the milder end of this spectrum.

FAS has three main components:
- Facial abnormalities
- Both intrauterine growth retardation and failure to catch up
- Cognitive impairment and learning disabilities

Alcohol dependence

Alcohol dependence, sometimes referred to as *alcohol addiction* or *alcoholism*, is defined in the International Classification of Mental and Behavioural Disorders (ICD-10) as a cluster of physiological, behavioural, and cognitive phenomena in which the use of a substance or class of substances takes on a much higher priority for a given individual than other behaviours (World Health Organisation, 1992). A diagnosis of alcohol dependence is commonly made if the individual has demonstrated three or more of the following criteria in the previous year:

- A strong desire or compulsion to consume alcohol, sometimes described as craving alcohol
- Difficulty in controlling consumption, may be associated with craving but also related to the difficulty in limiting drinking on a single occasion
- Physiological withdrawal state, commonly sweats, nausea, tremor, and, more seriously, seizures and dementia tremens
- Evidence of tolerance: the need to consume increasing amounts in order to achieve desired effects
- Progressive neglect of social and other activities, priority of drinking over family, employment, and other roles

In England, the prevalence of alcohol dependence was estimated to be 3.6% (6% of men and 2% of women) or about 1.1 million people. Regional variation in the prevalence of alcohol dependence was noted for the East Midlands (1.6%) region and in the North East and Yorkshire and Humber (5.2%) (Drummond et al., 2005). Based on 2006 data, it is estimated that alcohol dependence in Scotland is about 6%. The higher prevalence rate for alcohol dependence in Scotland is largely accounted for by the higher prevalence in men (6.7%) but particularly in women (3.3%) when compared to England (Drummond et al., 2009; SMACAP, 2011).

Mental health comorbidity

Comorbidity, or dual diagnosis, refers to the co-occurrence of harmful drinking, including alcohol dependence, and mental health problems (mental illness) in an individual at a particular point in his or her life. Community surveys conducted by Jenkins et al. (1997) reported a strong positive correlation between mental health symptoms and alcohol use; as mental health symptoms increase, so does substance use. There are a number of different ways in which the relationship between alcohol and mental illness can be explained, which depend on the level of alcohol consumption and the specific mental health condition. Individuals may use substances such as alcohol and illegal drugs to limit the negative aspects of mental illnesses, such as anxiety and depression. Conversely, heavy alcohol consumption can result in anxiety and depression as well as specific conditions associated with alcohol consumption, such as alcohol-related brain damage and Wernike–Korsakoff syndrome (MacLean, 2012).

In specialist alcohol services, the prevalence of mental health conditions was significant: affective and anxiety disorders, 81%; personality disorder, 53%; schizophrenia, 3%. In community and mental health services, 44% of service users reported a problem with alcohol or illicit drugs in the previous year (Weaver et al., 2003). Harmful and dependent drinking are also common features in patients of mental health services. Furthermore, high levels of prevalence of comorbidity are also noted in both prison and homeless populations (Scottish Government, 2003).

Alcohol-related deaths

In the UK, the term *alcohol-related deaths* refers to the underlying cause of death, the condition that initiated the events leading to death. Instances where alcohol is a contributory factor but not recorded as the underlying cause of death are excluded. This measure substantially underestimates the impact of alcohol on mortality. However, a broader definition includes any mention of alcohol on a death certificate. When conditions wholly attributable and partly attributable to alcohol are included in estimating the impact of alcohol and morbidity, the picture changes significantly.

In Northern Ireland in 2010, there were 284 alcohol-related deaths, an increase of 50% over the preceding decade (DoHSSPSNI, 2011). Alcohol accounted for 1000 deaths in Wales in 2009 (Alcohol Concern, 2010a,b). In Scotland in 2009, 53,856 deaths were recorded and 1282 (2.4%) of those deaths were instances where alcohol was the underlying cause. By considering 'any cause' by alcohol or 'any mention' of alcohol on death certificates, deaths attributable to alcohol virtually double, for example, Wales 2000, Scotland 2564, England (Jones

attributable fractions), and Northern Ireland 568 in 2009–2010.

In Scotland, 17.5% of all deaths in 16–24-year-old men were attributable to alcohol (ISD, 2011). Among those below the age of 35, the acute consequences of intoxication, including intentional self harm and traffic accidents, were the main causes of death. In contrast, those over the age of 35 were more commonly affected by the chronic health consequences of alcohol consumption (Jones et al., 2008; ISD, 2011). In 2009, more than two-thirds of the alcohol-related deaths were of people over 50 years of age, the same for both men and women. The death rate for men of all ages where alcohol is an underlying cause is double that for women (ISD, 2011). People living in urban areas in England and Wales experienced higher alcohol-related mortality compared to those living in rural areas, and there were also higher rates among those living in deprived circumstances (Erskine et al., 2010).

With regard to inequality and deprivation, rates of alcohol-related deaths ranged from 7.8 times greater in 2008 to 6.3 times greater in 2009 for the most deprived compared to the least deprived. In 2007, the alcohol-related mortality rate was almost double in Scotland compared to Wales (Gartner, 2009). In Northern Ireland, people living in the most deprived areas were five times more likely to die from an alcohol-related cause than those in the least deprived areas (DHSSPSNI, 2011).

The link between deprivation and alcohol harm

Health inequalities are an outcome of deprivation and poverty (Department of Health, 1998; Scottish Government, 2008a,b). Virtually every health measure associated with alcohol demonstrates a poorer outcome for those most deprived compared to the most affluent. Poor alcohol-related health markers and outcomes are not necessarily caused by greater alcohol consumption of those in lower socio-economic groups than those who are more affluent. The reverse is the case; see Chapter 1.

Those most deprived were around 4.5 times more likely to have primary health care contact (GP, health centre services) compared to those least deprived (ISD, 2011). The rate of hospital discharge from deprived areas was nine times that of more affluent areas (ISD, 2011). In England, three times as many deaths from alcoholic liver disease are recorded in the most deprived areas compared to the most affluent (Effiong et al., 2012).

Alcohol-related emergency hospital admissions rates for 1996–1997 and 2003–2004 are listed in Table 2.3; this table lists the most common alcohol-related emergency conditions. Substantial increases in rates of emergency admissions (per 10,000 of the population) are apparent for the period, for both men and women, including a 100% increase in the rate of emergency admissions for chronic liver disease among women and a 96% increase in the rate of emergency admissions for chronic pancreatitis among men. Increased alcohol-related emergency admissions during this period mirrored the increase in both alcohol sales and reported consumption during the same period. The percentage increase in emergency admissions for these conditions, irrespective of gender, is striking. As with other alcohol-related consequences, admissions increase significantly among those who are most deprived. Those most deprived were seven times more likely to be admitted as an emergency for acute alcohol intoxication, six times for liver disease, and eight times for chronic pancreatitis, whether male or female.

Box 2.3 reflects the increase in alcohol consumption in the general population during that period and the resultant alcohol-related consequences in conjunction with the impact of deprivation.

> ! **Thinking Point**
>
> Deprivation accounts for health inequalities reflected in alcohol-related health harm statistics in the UK but not completely. Why do you think this is?

Alcohol and offending

Despite public and policy concerns about binge drinking, drunkenness offences in the UK and Scotland have declined by 20% between 1998/1999 and 2007/2008 (ISD, 2011). It is possible that this may be because of altered police practices

Table 2.3 Emergency admission rates for alcohol-related conditions: 1996–1997 to 2003–2004: rates of increase (%) and deprivation comparisons: Scotland

ALCOHOL-RELATED CONDITION	INCREASE (%) IN RATE PER 10,000: 1996–1997 TO 2003–2004	DEPRIVATION: MOST DEPRIVED COMPARED TO LEAST DEPRIVED
Acute intoxication		
Males	40	7-fold increase in admissions
Females	30	(male and female)
Liver disease		
Males	71	More than 6-fold increase in admissions
Females	83	(male and female)
Chronic liver disease		
Males	92	2.7-fold increase in admissions
Females	100	(male and female)
Chronic pancreatitis		
Males	96	8-fold increase in admissions
Females	55	(male and female)
Oesophageal varices		
Males	50	3-fold increase in admissions
Females	33	(male and female)

Source: http://www.indicators.scot.nhs.uk/Reports/2005_Clinical_Indicators_Report.pdf, accessed 13/08/13.

brought about by the practicalities of policing large numbers of intoxicated people. Alcohol is involved in a wide range of offences where the alcohol consumption is not recorded in published statistics. However, it is broadly recognised that alcohol is involved in more than 50% of assaults and breaches of the peace. While most alcohol-related offending may be described as 'nuisance', there is also a strong association with serious offences, including serious assault and homicide.

The relationship between alcohol and offending

Alcohol is not criminogenic, that is, it does not cause crime. If it did cause crime, then all alcohol consumers would offend or behave badly. Clearly, they do not. However, alcohol and crime appear to be associated at a population level. There

---

Box 2.3 The Scottish/Glasgow effect

Deprivation is a fundamental determinant of health. The so-called 'Glasgow effect' refers to the higher levels of mortality and morbidity experienced in the deprived post-industrial region of West Central Scotland, with Glasgow at its centre, which exceeds that which may be explained by deprivation alone (Hanlon et al., 2006; Bromley and Shelton, 2010; McCartney et al., 2011). These measures are so significant that they skew the overall picture of Scotland's health. The 'Glasgow effect' reflects a slower rate of health improvement in the city compared to the rest of the UK, a phenomenon which may date from the early 1980s. A similar effect has also been reported in parts of both South Wales and North East England (Bromley and Shelton, 2010).

Glasgow, Manchester, and Liverpool, cities with almost identical deprivation profiles, have been compared. Gray (2007) noted that alcohol consumption was greater in Glasgow than the rest of Scotland. For the period 2003–2007, standardised all-cause mortality ratio comparisons demonstrated that, in Glasgow, there were 30% more premature deaths, with all deaths 15% higher than would be expected given the similarity in deprivation profiles among the three cities. In more deprived areas of Glasgow, premature deaths tended to be higher, particularly among males, and about half of these 'excess' deaths in those under age 65 were directly attributable to alcohol (32%) and drugs (17%) (Hanlon et al., 2006).

Alcohol-related causes of death were 2.3 times greater in Glasgow than in Liverpool and Manchester and, similarly, drug-related deaths (in which alcohol is also implicated) were 2.5 times greater.

While there are many theories that seek to explain these phenomena, there is a general acceptance that substance use, and alcohol in particular, plays a significant part in the 'Glasgow effect', even in other areas of the UK (McCartney et al., 2011).

---

are a number of important associations, and many offenders and victims have alcohol in their blood at the time of the offence. A direct link between alcohol and crime implies that the offence would not have occurred in the absence of alcohol. The Home Office (2004) defined alcohol-related crime as instances of crime and disorder that occurred, and occurred at that level of seriousness, because alcohol consumption was a contributory factor. The nature of alcohol's contribution to offending varies. Alcohol consumption may indirectly affect crime in the following ways:

- Crime in order to access or afford alcohol
- Alcohol problems produce a home environment conducive to crime and antisocial behaviour
- Alcohol facilitates crime in individuals with low impulse control
- Alcohol triggers or facilitates aggression

- Alcohol has a negative impact on inhibition, judgement and decision making
- Some offences may be recorded because the offender is too drunk to escape
- Drunks may be easily victimised
- Alcohol is a scapegoat or excuse for bad behaviour

As alcohol is widely available in the UK and alcohol-related offending is concerned with conduct 'under the influence', one must understand the individual and environmental or contextual factors (see Chapter 1). In contrast, in the case of illicit drugs, prohibition dictates that the main offences relate to possession or supply of drugs or acquisitive crime to fund a drug habit rather than conduct under the influence.

Costs of alcohol-related offending

Approximately 44% of all violent offences are committed by individuals under the influence of alcohol (British Crime Survey 2010/2011). In the UK, it is estimated that the total cost of crime associated with alcohol is between £8 billion and £13 billion annually, at 2003 prices (Ministry of Justice, 2012; http://www.justice.gov.uk/downloads/legislation/bills-acts/legal-aid-sentencing/laspo-sobriety-ia.pdf).

The Scottish government estimates the 2007 costs of alcohol-related crime were £727 million, accounting for 20% of the total overall costs of alcohol misuse. Around 75% of the costs associated with alcohol and offending result from a consequence of the crimes, while 20% of the costs are costs of the criminal justice system (police, courts, probation services, and prison) (Beale et al., 2009).

Criminal justice systems

There is no single criminal justice system in the UK. The criminal justice systems of Northern Ireland and Scotland are distinct from each other and also different from those of England and Wales. One feature of this diversity is that what constitutes an alcohol-related offence may be different in each country. In turn, the responses to the same offence may also be quite different. However, there are also some important similarities in the ways in which alcohol-related offending is handled. First, some offences where alcohol plays a significant part are not recorded or recognised as alcohol-related offences (e.g. alcohol features heavily in charges of 'assault', but it is not recorded as 'alcohol-related assault'). Second, there is a distinction between civil offences, where the offence is defined by local bye-laws (e.g. breach of the peace (Scotland), drinking in public or restricted areas), and criminal offences. While very common, civil offences are minor offences. More serious offences (assault, murder) are dealt with by the courts and criminal justice systems, which can impose more severe penalties for these more serious offences.

Civil offences

It is important to note that, in an era of increased alcohol consumption, there has been a proliferation of legal responses designed to deter drunkenness and punish the intoxicated individual. This is seen more generally as a move towards criminalising antisocial behaviour in the UK (Rodger, 2008).

Place, possession, and consumption

Some offences relate to the possession and/or consumption of alcohol in certain places and do not necessarily imply drunkenness or any particular offensive behaviour. In certain locations, drinking or possession of alcohol is an offence. Since the early 1990s, local authorities have had the power to introduce bye-laws that ban drinking alcohol in particular 'designated places' (e.g. in towns or town and city centres) to prevent or limit alcohol-fuelled public disorder: 'Any person who consumes alcoholic liquor in a designated place or is found to be in possession of an open container in a designated place shall be guilty of an offence'.

The offence is essentially possession and/or consumption, not drunkenness. The rise in offences is explained by the enactment of such a bye-law rather than an increase in offending. Significant increases in these offences reflect the gradual implementation of such bye-laws by local authorities across the UK.

Possession of alcohol is banned by law in sports grounds in Scotland.

Sobering-up services: Drunk and incapable

The term *drunk and incapable* refers to persons who are intoxicated to such a level that it is impossible for them to look after themselves. In addition to dealing with alcohol-fuelled antisocial behaviour, police services have also to deal with those who are drunk and incapable. Under the Criminal Justice (Scotland) Act 1980, 'designated places' for sobering up are defined as '. . . place[s] suitable for the care of drunken persons', where individuals are taken by police. Service users include those who are drunk on a single occasion and never make contact with a sobering-up service again, so-called *binge drinkers* who present on several occasions, and 'chronic recidivists' who are likely to be alcohol dependent and will present on numerous occasions. The practices involved in the delivery of sobering-up services vary greatly across the UK; most have designated places for sobering up, have a base, and operate 7 days a week. In many parts of the UK, the services may include triage, first aid, custody nurses, cell monitoring, ambulance and police protocols, accident and emergency services, and mobile services in city centre hotspots (Griesbach et al., 2009).

In the absence of formal sobering-up services, the burden falls to police and NHS accident and emergency staff. In

Scotland in 2006–2007, the costs of holding drunk and incapable individuals in police cells were £2.12 million. This group's impact on health services during the same period was estimated to be between £0.7 million and £1.95 million. Use of accident and emergency services by this group cost £93 per hospital visit, with a further cost of £0.7 million for acute hospital beds at a cost of £483 per bed per day (Griesbach et al., 2009).

Fixed-penalty notice

The introduction of fixed-penalty notices (FPNs) in Scotland was designed to enable police to deal with antisocial behaviours more effectively, particularly during night-time drinking hours, and is consistent with the recommendation to prioritise police attention to nuisance behaviours, especially around licensed premises (Scottish Executive, 2004). An FPN is viewed as providing police with a course of action proportionate to the offence, while maintaining police presence on the street.

A large proportion of FPNs issued in Scotland from 2007 to 2009 – around 62,000 of a total of 65,000 – were used for three main offences, all related to alcohol-related nuisance: 'breach of the peace', 'drinking alcohol in public', and 'urinating and defecating in public' (Scottish Government, 2009).

In a survey of police officers, 80% considered that most of the people given FPNs were under the influence of alcohol, commonly around licensed premises and town and city centres, including public transport settings. Police officers interviewed were divided on whether FPNs would result in a long-term reduction in antisocial behaviour (Scottish Government, 2009).

Drink-banning orders

Drink-banning orders (DBOs) are civil orders, similar to antisocial behaviour orders, which can last from 2 months to 2 years. They are available through the provisions of the Violent Crime Reduction Act (2006) and have been available on application in England and Wales since 2009.

A DBO can be made against a person age 16 or over if they engage in criminal or disorderly conduct while under the influence of alcohol and the court considers it necessary to protect the public from their behaviour.

DBOs are individualised and may impose any prohibition which the court considers necessary to protect others from alcohol-related crime or disorderly conduct committed under the influence of alcohol. These schemes involve alcohol abstinence and monitoring that require the offender to abstain from drinking for a set period as part of an attempt to reduce alcohol-related crime. Such an intervention within the criminal justice system seeks to ensure robust and demanding consequences for drinking and committing crime, deter offenders from committing further alcohol-related crime, and increase public safety. An impact assessment of compulsory abstinence concluded that it is not known whether it will reduce offending (Ministry of Justice, 2012).

Violence and homicide

Substance misuse contributes to the majority of homicides in England and Wales. A 3-year national clinical survey identified 1594 homicide perpetrators: 42% of perpetrators had a history of alcohol problems or dependence, and 40% had a history of drug misuse or dependence. Alcohol played a major role in 6% and a minor role in 39% of homicides, while drugs played a major role in 1% and a minor role in 14% of homicides. Alcohol- and drug-related homicides were generally associated with male perpetrators who had a history of violence, personality disorders, mental health service contact, and with victims unknown to the perpetrator (Shaw et al., 2006).

In Scotland in 2009–2010, 65% of those accused of homicide were under the influence of alcohol or drugs (Box 2.4).

Box 2.4 Murder in private

Strathclyde Police, comparing April to November 2010 with the same period in 2009, reported a 73% increase in murders, which represents 4.4% increase of the average for the previous 5 years. Such an increase contradicted the significant downward trends in attempted murder (29%), serious assaults (26%), and common assaults (9%).

The police concluded that, of the 40 homicides recorded from April to November 2010, 60% occurred in private places. Thus, murders increased in places most difficult to police: the home or a private place. The key factors involved appear to be:

Cheap alcohol bought from off-licences or supermarkets rather than the more expensive licensed premises

Private drinking parties that take place inside and thus are hidden from the gaze of the police, who normally react robustly to street disorder and violence

Drinking and drink-fuelled violence in private is more dangerous than in a pub (publicans are duty bound to respond to drunkenness) or a public place. In the latter, there are greater controls on behaviour and a greater likelihood that emergency services would be called by a sober individual.

At a heavy drinking party, drunken participants may not react to control the risky behaviour of others and perhaps fail to act quickly enough when violence occurs.

Consequently, 70% of all murder victims attacked in private settings die at the scene. The opposite is the case for those hurt in public, and they tend to lose their lives in hospital, while a majority survive.

Source: Leask (2010).

In the UK, in 63% of incidents of wounding, 55% of assaults with minor injury, and 50% of assaults without injury, victims believed offenders were under the influence of alcohol. This view was more common among male than female victims as well as among younger than older victims and was a consistent finding in England, Wales, and Scotland. Almost half of younger victims were also under the influence of alcohol at the time they were attacked (Fitzpatrick and Thorne, 2010; ISD, 2011).

Domestic violence

Alcohol is estimated to be consumed before 73% of domestic violence incidents, while 48% of those convicted of domestic violence are dependent on alcohol (Gilchrist et al., 2003; Fitzpatrick and Thorne, 2010; Galvani, 2010). Further detail about the association between domestic violence and alcohol can be found in Chapter 5.

Drink driving: Law and health

The Road Traffic Act 1967 introduced the drink-driving legal limit of 80 mg of alcohol per 100 ml of blood (or 35 mg of alcohol per 100 ml of breath) in the UK; most other EU countries have lower limits, Luxembourg and Ireland being exceptions. Alcohol affects driving skills (coordination, judgement, risk awareness) at low levels of consumption, certainly well below the legal limit in the UK. In the first 7 years after the Road Traffic Act, an estimated 5000 alcohol-related deaths

and 200,000 alcohol-related crashes were prevented (Dunbar, 1992).

The prevalence of drinking (any alcohol) and driving has decreased since 2001 both in terms of a person ever having driven after drinking (from 55% to 43%, 2001–2007) and having done so in the previous year (from 37% to 35%, 2001–2007) (Collins et al., 2008; ISD, 2011).

Therefore, two populations of convicted drink drivers exist: young people who consume large amounts of alcohol and have relatively limited driving skills and harmful or problem drinkers who drive. In a study of alcohol-affected drivers, older drivers, including those who drive as part of their job, had higher liver enzyme measures (gamma glutamyl transferase, GGT), a measure of harmful drinking, which was associated with traffic accidents but not blood alcohol concentrations or previous convictions (Dunbar, 1992).

There are distinctions in occupational backgrounds, whereby those in manual and skill-manual occupations have significantly higher drink-driving conviction rates than those in professional occupations, including school students. The car insurance industry indicates that there are pockets of society that have a higher proportion of drink-driving convictions than others. It might not be surprising to see that this is largely male dominated, and the professions with the higher proportion of convictions are therefore skewed towards the more male-dominated, blue-collar workforces.

Drink-driving convictions also show significant regional variation across the UK. Analysis of the data by geographic location shows that the highest proportion of drink or drug-related convictions per motor insurance quote is in South Wales with 6.7 convictions per 1000 quotations, followed by North Scotland at 6.4 and Mid Wales at 5.9 per 1000 insurance claims. These findings indicate more about police practice than alcohol consumption in these areas. In areas of deprivation, a low level of car ownership will also reflect low drink-driving conviction rates (http://www.moneysupermarket.com/car-insurance/monitor-drink-driving-convictions/, accessed 11/09/13).

Drink-driving offences in the UK have fluctuated since 2000 with a downward trend. There may be several reasons for this, including public health drink-driving campaigns, the threat of being caught and convicted, and increased motoring and insurance premium costs.

In the UK, some methods of drink-driving prevention that have been demonstrated to be effective, such as random breath testing, sobriety checkpoints, a lowered legal limit (though this is the Scottish government's intention), and a lowered legal limit for younger drivers, are not used (Babor et al., 2003). The implementation of evidence-based methods is opposed by those with opposing perspectives.

Alcohol affects judgement and reaction time at blood/breath alcohol measures significantly below the legal limit (Box 2.5). Alan may drink less than he used to, which is consistent with many older people; however, he does drink regularly, both in company and alone. This combination is associated with drinking at hazardous levels, which, given his age, may have an impact on his driving skills. He has committed no offence. Emerging opinion suggests a recommended daily consumption limit of one unit of alcohol for older people (Health Scotland, 2006).

GGT indicates hazardous or harmful consumption of alcohol. While this is not an offence, the Driver and Vehicle Licensing Agency (DVLA) issues guidance on substance use issues that requires a GP to report such a finding and the driver to stop driving for 6 months minimum with a view to demonstrating a reduction in mean corpuscular volume (MCV) to within set norms. This may be viewed as a public health intervention and road accident prevention strategy; the underlying assumption is that alcohol consumption at a level which raises MCV implies an increased likelihood of driving while under the influence of alcohol (https://www.dvla.gov.uk/dvla/medical/aag/Chapterview/Drug%20and%20, accessed 11/09/2013).

Currently, a debate about reducing the legal limit for drink driving is being waged. The Scottish government has pressured

---

> ### ! Thinking Point
>
> Under what drink-driving circumstances should someone have their licence removed?

Box 2.5 Case study: Over what limit?

Alan is 84 years old and has been driving since his teens while working on farms and later as a lorry driver. He prides himself on his driving skills. He has been widowed for 10 years and is fiercely independent; he enjoys a drink most days, sometimes with friends and family, or on his own. His family joke with him that it's about time he stopped driving though they are increasingly concerned about his erratic driving and the potential for him to injure himself or others. Alan is adamant that he will stop driving when he's ready as he'll know when the time is right.

Alan reversed his car into a neighbour's car, causing substantial damage. The police were called and found Alan to be upset and unsteady on his feet and therefore decided to breathalyse him. He was just below the legal limit (60 mg/ 100 ml), and he was taken to the police station, where he was treated very kindly and retested. Again, he was below the legal limit. He was mystified by this incident and admitted that his memory of the event was hazy.

Some weeks later, his GP, as part of a routine health screening, asked Alan about his alcohol consumption and also took a blood sample. Alan's blood sample showed a raised GGT. The GP, suspicious about Alan's alcohol consumption, was duty bound to report the matter to the DVLA, and advised Alan to stop driving for 6 months or until his blood tests showed a result in the normal range.

---

the UK government and proposed a reduction in the drink-driving legal limit to 50 mg of alcohol per 100 ml of blood. Such a change would have resulted in a drink-driving conviction for Alan.

Criminal justice system disposals

The impact of alcohol may be seen both in the number and types of alcohol-related offences as well as the prevalence of alcohol issues in offender populations based on court disposal.

Arrest referral schemes

Arrest referral schemes are designed as early interventions that target alcohol-related offenders to offer brief advice or referral to further services. A Home Office review conducted in England focused on those over the age of 18 who had been arrested and were deemed to be under the influence of alcohol (excluding drink-driving offences). The review found that 35% were drinking hazardously, 11% were drinking harmfully, and 38% were dependent drinkers, the latter requiring more than alcohol brief interventions (ABI). More than half of those arrested for alcohol-related offences had not been arrested in the previous 6 months. This suggests that those arrested during night-time drinking hours were not regular offenders, despite their raised levels of alcohol consumption, thereby calling into question the efficacy of arrest referral. Almost two-thirds of arrests were for minor alcohol-related offences (drunk and disorderly, criminal damage, public order offences), and more than one-third were for violent offences (Blakeborough and Richardson, 2012).

Probation

A probation order consists of community-based support for, and supervision of, offenders and is conferred by a court. In a study of probationers, 44% had an alcohol problem, 48% were found to binge drink, 41% had displayed violent behaviour linked to alcohol use, and 48% had a criminogenic need directly related to alcohol misuse (Fitzpatrick and Thorne, 2010) (see Chapter 6 for details on ABIs within probation services).

Prison populations

In a review of substance use problems in prisons, estimates of the prevalence of alcohol problems and dependence ranged from 18% to 30% in male prisoners and from 10% to 24% in female prisoners (Fazel et al., 2006). In England, 63% of sentenced male prisoners and 39% of sentenced female prisoners admitted to hazardous drinking prior to imprisonment, of which about half were dependent on alcohol (Prison Reform Trust, 2004).

In Scottish prison populations, about 50% of prisoners (male and female) indicate that they were drunk at the time of the offence (ISD, 2011). There is a marked difference between young offenders (under 21 years of age) (77% of whom admit to being drunk at the time of the offence) compared to adult offenders (44% of whom admit to being drunk at the time of the offence). Screening the prison population in 2007 and 2009 resulted in just under half of the prison population being identified as having an alcohol problem (Macaskill et al., 2011).

 Summary Points

(1) Alcohol contributes very significantly to poor health and offending.
(2) Measures of alcohol-related consequences tend to rise and fall, mirroring alcohol sales data and self-reported alcohol consumption rates in surveys.
(3) Reductions in consumption in the UK as a whole are reflected in decreases in many alcohol-related consequences.
(4) Virtually every aspect of health care is impacted by the consumption of alcohol, ranging from emergency hospital admissions to chronic health consequences.
(5) Alcohol consumption also impacts psychiatric services, most of which is attributable to alcohol dependence and comorbidity.
(6) Similar impacts are reflected in alcohol-related offending, including drink-driving and violent offences.
(7) Both alcohol-related health consequences and offending impact families and communities.

Continued

(8) Most attention has been paid to public disorder as a consequence of binge drinking. As a result, the last 20 years have seen the emergence of a range of offences across the UK designed to curb this common drinking pattern, reduce public disorder, and maintain police presence.

(9) Alcohol use is implicated in more serious offences that include violence, domestic violence, and homicide. Consequently, there is a significant proportion of problem drinkers in probation and prison populations.

(10) Virtually every alcohol-related health indicator suggests that there is a greater impact on those who are less affluent.

(11) The significant costs associated with alcohol justify intervention to prevent harm and, in turn, reduce costs to health and criminal justice services.

Web pages and resources

http://www.alcoholconcern.org.uk/assets/files/Publications/Health%20impacts%20factsheet%20November%202010.pdf
A factsheet on the impact of alcohol on health, with up-to-date figures.

http://www.ncdalliance.org/alcohol
Read the briefing on why addressing harmful use of alcohol is essential to realising the goals of the UN resolution on noncommunicable diseases (NCDs).

http://www.publications.parliament.uk/pa/cm200910/cmselect/cmhealth/151/15107.htm
The impact of alcohol on health, the NHS, and society.

Further reading

Rehm, U., et al., 2009. Global burden of disease and injury and economic cost attributable to alcohol use and alcohol-use disorders. Lancet 373 (9682), 2223–2233.

The burden of mortality and disease attributable to alcohol is quantified, both globally and for 10 large countries. There is an assessment of alcohol exposure and prevalence of alcohol-use disorders on the basis of reviews of published work. Other major disease categories causally linked to alcohol are identified and an estimate made of attributable fractions by sex, age, and WHO region. Additionally, the social costs of alcohol are estimated in selected countries.

Rehm, J., Room, R., 2009. A case study in how harmful alcohol consumption can be. Lancet 373 (9682), 2176–2177.

In discussing a case study of how harmful to health widespread heavy drinking in a population can be, Rehm and Room examine the total impact that heavy alcohol drinking can have on society, including the many social problems and harm to people other than the drinker.

Shaw, J., Hunt, I.M., Flynn, S., Amos, T., Meehan, J., Robinson, J., Bickley, H., Parsons, R., McCann, K., Burns, J., Kapur, N., Appleby, L., 2006. The role of alcohol and drugs in homicides in England and Wales. Addiction 101.

This paper provides a detailed outline of alcohol, drugs, and homicide, with focus on the characteristics of perpetrators.

3 Dependent drinkers and recovery

Recovery requires behavioural adjustment, irrespective of whether treatment is part of that process. A significant majority of individuals who develop substance-related problems change their behaviour without formal intervention or treatment (Klingemann, 2004). Some view treatment as simply the skilful nudge towards and support for self-determined change (Edwards, 2000).

This chapter emphasises the fundamental nature of behavioural change and considers the role and effectiveness of treatment within that process. Evidence of personal resources or recovery capital required to achieve behaviour change and maintain recovery is explored. The idiosyncratic nature of change and recovery will be examined, as will the role of mutual self-help, including "12-step" approaches.

The characteristics of people who seek treatment are identified and considered in relation to treatment outcomes and recovery capital. The research that underpins current evidence-based practice is evaluated by exploring reviews of specialist alcohol treatment studies and client-treatment matching studies. The similarities in outcome from different treatment interventions, which point to common change processes, are explored.

Definitions and terminology

The subject of change and recovery has a long history and over time a wide range of terms have been used, reflecting different cultural values. A number of terms refer to the process of changing behaviour without formal help or treatment, including "self-change", "unassisted/ unaided change", "self-quitter", "natural recovery," and "spontaneous remission". These terms are used interchangeably in the literature.

Definitions of recovery vary and are dependent on country and culture of origin. The Scottish Ministerial Advisory Committee on Alcohol Problems (SMACAP) points to the long history of the recovery movement, which goes back at least 150 years. Its nature has changed significantly over this time, responding to shifts in the way that society has conceived and prioritised alcohol problems. It is an evolving concept, but, in general, recovery is taken to mean the process through which an individual is enabled to move on from problematic alcohol use towards a life free of alcohol-related problems, and this individual is then able to become an active and contributing member of the society (SMACAP, 2011). In contrast, the Betty Ford Institute Consensus Panel (BFICP, 2007) defines recovery as a voluntarily maintained lifestyle characterised by sobriety, personal health and citizenship. Further, dimensions of recovery include remission of the substance use disorder, enhancement in health (physical, emotional, relational, occupational and spiritual), and positive community inclusion (White, 2007).

The last two definitions reflect an American perspective, where there is a stronger attachment to "12-Step" approaches and abstinence is a key element in the recovery journey. Consequently, these definitions are more prescriptive than that offered by SMACAP, which states that a recovery ethos supports and builds on individual strengths and assets, thus enabling individuals to move from harmful drinking to a life free of alcohol-related problems. However, none of these definitions necessarily prescribe the methods that should be implemented to achieve recovery.

Recovery capital refers to the quantity and quality of resources, both internal and external, that can be used to initiate and sustain recovery (Laudet and White, 2008); this term is synonymous with social capital (Granfield and Cloud, 1999). Having a high level of recovery capital is a positive treatment-outcome predictor.

Treatment is regarded as a time-limited, circumscribed experience that interacts with and, hopefully, enhances the self-change process on the road to recovery (Di Clemente, 2006).

A model of change

The most prominent model of change is "stages in the process of change" or the transtheoretical model (TTM), which serves as an important function in providing a common language across disciplines involved in health behaviours (see Box 3.1). The early research that informed this model was based on smokers who were self-quitters and not treatment attenders. The model indicates that there are distinct stages in making changes as well as distinct change processes, which are evident to a greater or lesser degree in each stage (Prochaska and Di Clemente, 1983).

The TTM also outlines processes that are described as the engines of change (Di Clemente and Prochaska, 1998), with or without formal treatment. The model cuts across the artificial distinction between self-changers and treatment seekers (see Table 3.1).

Box 3.1 TTM stages

Precontemplation: The individual is not considering changing drinking behaviour and will identify the positive aspects of their drinking, though often coerced into services by employers, family, or the criminal justice system.

Contemplation: The drinker considers the pros and cons of drinking and change. For some, this may be a period of considerable inner conflict and also of considerable duration.

Preparation: The drinker makes a commitment and plans for imminent action to change.

Action: The drinker is actively involved in changing his or her behaviour and in engaging the required resources to support this change and prevent relapse.

Maintenance: The drinker achieves this stage about 6 months after "quitting", or changing behaviour, when new behaviours are established and reinforced by supportive influences. This would be described as early recovery (Best et al., 2010).

Source: Prochaska and Di Clemente (1983).

Table 3.1 Change processes

CHANGE PROCESSES	EXAMPLE
Cognitive	
Consciousness raising[a]	Look for information on alcohol
Self-liberation[a]	Self-talk on ability to stop
Social liberation	Aware of options for non-drinking
Self re-evaluation	Disappointment at continued heavy drinking
Environmental re-evaluation	Negative impact of alcohol on the environment
Dramatic relief	Emotional response to health warnings or portrayals of drinking problems
Behavioural	
Counter-conditioning	Engage in alternative activities
Stimulus control	Remove things from environment or avoidance (e.g. avoiding the pub and friends who drink heavily)
Reinforcement management	Plan rewards: reinforcement from others for moderation or abstinence
Helping relationships[a]	Having someone who listens

[a]*Most commonly used processes.*

Cognitive processes are evident among those individuals in the Contemplation and Preparation stages, while behavioural processes are more commonly used in the Action and Maintenance stages. However, the most commonly used processes are consciousness-raising, self-liberation, and helping relationships. These are very general change processes and not specific to alcohol problems in particular. Orford (2001) suggests that information about cognitive and behavioural processes assists us in explaining why it is that treatment with very different rationales, or indeed no treatment at all, may allow the same fundamental processes to take place.

! Thinking Point

(1) Why do you think consciousness-raising, self-liberation, and helping relationships are the most commonly used processes?

(2) What do you think might be potential barriers to changing alcohol-related behaviour?

Self-change and recovery

In an epidemiological survey of 43,093 US adults, researchers investigated the probability of remission from nicotine, alcohol, cannabis and cocaine dependence. A significant proportion of dependent people stopped, with rates for alcohol and tobacco around 90%, and rates for cannabis and cocaine between 97% and 99%. This indicates the relative difficulty that individuals experience in giving up or cutting down their use of substances that are socially accepted and easily available. Lower remission rates were also associated with mental health issues, indicating that self-change may also be more difficult for some on the basis of their life circumstances (Lopez-Quintero et al., 2011). A survey conducted in Clydebank identified 160 individuals who met the criteria of former problem drinkers. When asked about the reasons for changing their drinking, family relationships, employment, finances and health were the most commonly reported influences on drinking behaviour and only those with the most severe alcohol problems reported treatment (Saunders and Kershaw, 1979). These reasons are commonly reported in studies of both self-changers and treatment-attenders and also predict treatment outcomes (Orford and Edwards, 1977).

In a study of 30 heroin and 30 alcohol self-changers (Klingemann, 2004), it was reported that they generally went through a conscious phase of preliminary deliberation, reflecting on life events that were experienced negatively in the previous year, which in turn progressed to more serious motivation for change. Spontaneous remitters used distancing or avoidance techniques (avoiding the pub or heavy drinking friends, or taking a different route home), substitution of alcohol, negative expectancy (the belief that bad things will happen if drinking is resumed), and behaviour management (alternative activities and hobbies) in the early stages of their recovery. Motivation to change implies that the good things about drinking are outweighed by the bad and that something needs to be done about it. These current concerns are considered to be cognitive elements that influence decisions to change (Cox and Klinger, 2004). An absence of current concerns would suggest that change was unlikely. Natural recovery appears more difficult for problem drinkers than illicit drug users, as ex-drinkers (or controlled drinkers) continue to be confronted by high-risk situations and the easy availability of alcohol, whereas illicit drug use is less culturally accepted and integrated (Klingemann, 2004; Lopez-Quintero et al., 2011).

Three distinct groups of self-changers were identified in a media recruitment study: (Bischof et al., 2003):

- High severity of alcohol dependence, low alcohol-related problems, and low social support
- High severity of alcohol dependence, high alcohol-related problems, and medium social support
- Low severity of alcohol dependence, low alcohol-related problems, late onset, and high social support

Identifying the heterogeneity of self-changers and specific subgroups allows consideration of differences in initiation and maintenance of change or recovery. Further, the idea that self-changers are not "real alcoholics" is contradicted by these findings, in relation to the high severity of alcohol dependence.

Rumpf et al. (2000) compared 176 media-recruited alcohol-dependent self-changers, with 32 derived from a representative general population. Those recruited via the media were more likely to have abstained from drinking alcohol in the previous 12 months, be more severely dependent, and have greater prior health and social problems. They experienced greater social pressure to change and reported less life satisfaction prior to changing.

In a study of paths to recovery, over 400 inner-city males were followed from age 14 to age 47. At follow-up, 110 of the men met the criteria for "alcohol abuse", and just under half had achieved at least one year of abstinence. Stable abstinence was associated with greater severity of alcohol abuse or dependence, finding "substitute dependencies", new relationships, behaviour modification, and engagement with Alcoholics Anonymous (AA) or a religious group. It was concluded that neither treatment nor good pre-morbid adjustment were predictive of abstinence. Less than one in five were able to successfully return to problem-free drinking, having had fewer symptoms of dependence and alcohol-related problems (Vaillant and Milofsky, 1982).

Further follow-up after 60 years found the cohort more than 70 years old, and, of those contacted, 32% were abstinent and 1% were controlled drinkers. A further 12% were abusing alcohol, and it was noted that this pattern of consumption persisted for decades, without remission, death, or progression to severe dependence: chronic dependence was rare. Consistent with earlier findings, sustained abstinence was best predicted by prior dependence on alcohol and AA attendance (Vaillant, 2003).

Mutual self-help

It has long been known that groups have a powerful influence on shaping and supporting behaviour (Barrie, 1990). Self-help group members perceive themselves to share a common problem and support each other in its resolution. Groups are led by those who have achieved their status by their efforts at resolving their own problems while actively supporting the efforts of others. In self-help groups, support, goal direction, group norms, role models, involvement in alternative rewarding activities, teaching and developing coping skills, and supporting self-efficacy are some of the ingredients responsible for a positive impact (Moos, 2008). However, 12-step groups and agencies are quite distinct. Cornerstones of 12-step teaching are spirituality in the acceptance of a higher power and active promulgation of the view that alcoholism is a disease, which can only be arrested by abstinence. Thus, 12-step programmes are based on a belief system; it has been suggested in the past that AA is a cult (Bufe, 1998).

However, "12-Step" is the most widely known self-help approach, worldwide as well as in the UK, encompassing groups such as Alcoholics Anonymous (Box 3.2),

Al-Anon (for family members), Alateen (for children and young people whose parent(s) have an alcohol problem). Other associated 12-step approaches are Minnesota (a residential 12-step intervention), Hazeleden, and 12-step facilitation (TSF), which is designed to increase access to and engagement in AA.

Once introduced by their sponsor, a new member can expect the support of other group members in achieving and maintaining abstinence from alcohol on the basis of mutuality among equals. Regular attendance enables the individual to interact in a supportive non-drinking environment, where mutual reinforcement of attendance and sobriety are key features. AA members are recovering alcoholics, not recovered.

Mutual self-help as a preferred option

A significant number of those recovering from alcohol problems attend AA without ever attending formal treatment services. In a 3-year longitudinal follow-up study, two paths out of drinking problems were noted (Humphreys et al., 1995). Almost half of the subjects became moderate drinkers or stably abstinent. Those who subsequently became abstinent were of low socio-economic status, had severe drinking problems, and believed their drinking was a very serious problem. Once they began their recovery, they relied heavily on AA support. By contrast, the moderate drinkers had higher socio-economic status as well as

---

Box 3.2 The AA 12 steps (the same steps apply to Narcotics Anonymous, NA)

1. We admitted we were powerless over alcohol – that our lives had become unmanageable.
2. We came to believe that a Power greater than ourselves could restore us to sanity.
3. We made a decision to turn our will and our lives over to the care of God as we understood Him.
4. We made a searching and fearless moral inventory of ourselves.
5. We admitted to God, to ourselves, and to another human being the exact nature of our wrongs.
6. We were entirely ready to have God remove all these defects of character.
7. We humbly asked Him to remove our shortcomings.
8. We made a list of all persons we had harmed and became willing to make amends to them all.
9. We made direct amends to such people wherever possible, except when to do so would injure them or others.
10. We continued to take personal inventory and, when we were wrong, promptly admitted it.
11. We sought through prayer and meditation to improve our conscious contact with God as we understood Him, praying only for knowledge of His will for us and the power to carry that out.
12. Having had a spiritual awakening as the result of these steps, we tried to carry this message to alcoholics and to practice these principles in all our affairs.

Source: http://www.alcoholics-anonymous.org.uk/About-AA/The-12-Steps-of-AA (accessed 02/08/2013).

---

social support, and, hence, recovery capital. Paradoxically, it is also widely recognised that AA meetings are held exclusively for high status groups and professions, such as doctors, police, lawyers.

Few studies on natural recovery have considered the role of maintenance factors relevant to staying alcohol free. Self-help group attenders informed more people than non-attenders about their former alcohol problems, which resulted in reinforcement for their efforts, including support in coping with craving, thus increasing their social engagement and helping to sustain their recovery (Bischof et al., 2000).

12-step as an adjunct and follow-up to treatment

In the USA, AA-only and outpatient groups achieved similar effectiveness and demonstrated an improvement on no treatment (Humphreys and Moos, 1996; Ouimette et al., 1998). In the UK, as part of the National Treatment-Outcome

Research Study (NTORS), a follow-up study on treated problem drug users, the impact of Narcotics Anonymous (NA) and AA at a 5-year follow-up was investigated. Of those in residential treatment (or rehabilitation), where there was an emphasis on abstinence, abstinence from opiates and alcohol was greater at 5 years, compared to pre-treatment levels. Those who attended AA/NA after treatment, and did so more frequently, were more likely to be abstinent from alcohol and drugs. It was concluded that AA/NA can support and supplement residential treatment as an aftercare resource (Gossop et al., 2008). Similar conclusions were reached in studies in the USA (Fiorentine, 1999; Kaskutas et al., 2005).

Inpatient treatment attenders were followed up for 6 months in the UK. Frequent AA attenders had superior drinking outcomes (reduced drinking, fewer alcohol-related problems, and more abstinent days) compared to infrequent and non-AA attenders. The role of AA as a useful aftercare resource was confirmed. Despite these improvements, many individuals in the sample had alcohol and psychiatric problems at follow-up (Gossop et al., 2003).

Therefore, 12-step approaches are shown to be an effective support for recovery subsequent to treatment for alcohol problems. There are more than 3000 AA meetings per week in the UK, with around 500 taking place in London (Harris et al., 2003). Consequently, AA provides easy access to support groups in urban areas. However, there have been detractors who argue that AA is unscientific, smacks of fundamentalist religion, excludes those who do not espouse its views, and is not open to other forms of help for alcoholics (Vaillant, 1983).

! Thinking Point

(1) Is mutual self-help appropriate or necessary for all problem drinkers?
(2) How important do you think a non-drinking environment is to recovery?

Individual recovery paths

Paths to recovery are idiosyncratic, reflecting the circumstances leading up to a decision to change and the support available, including treatment for some. Recovery is essentially the story of each individual's personal journey into abuse or dependence and the path they take in finding a way out (Di Clemente, 2006). This is described in the two case studies in Box 3.3.

It cannot be assumed that both individuals described in Box 3.3 have a similar motivation or belief in their own ability to change; however, the following themes are relevant.

1. The individuals' life experiences and current alcohol-related problems are very different. Both gender and social background play a part, and the only common theme is that

---

Box 3.3 Case studies

Recovery no. 1

John is 28 years old and had a troubled family background that resulted in him spending some of his teenage years in care, during which time his drinking and disruptive behaviour became a source of concern. His father had an alcohol problem. Though considered able, he left school without qualifications. John has little contact with members of his family, and these few meetings have often been acrimonious. Subsequently, he didn't settle and has spent a significant amount of time homeless or in prison for violent offences that occurred when drunk and failure to pay fines for other alcohol-related offences. While in prison, he has participated in alcohol-information sessions; however, on liberation, he has frequently reoffended. John seldom makes contact with helping services when released from prison, other than homeless accommodation. He has worked occasionally as a labourer, usually away from his home area, and these periods are marked by periods of harm-free drinking and abstinence. John describes these times as feeling like he was "getting on track".

His heavy drinking and lifestyle have resulted in John experiencing poor health for a man of his age. He reports symptoms of alcohol dependence, and he binge drinks for days at a time, or until his money, or that of his drinking colleagues, runs out. He is in the early stages of liver damage and may be depressed.

Recovery no. 2

Janice is 40 years old. She runs her own small business and is a lone parent, having separated from her long-term partner, who was also her business partner, 3 years ago. She comes from a supportive family and describes her teenage drinking as "just like the rest of the girls". Her parents, who live nearby, are very involved in the care of her 7-year-old son and are concerned about their daughter's work situation.

Her café/bar business is in financial difficulty and may have to be sold. This difficulty may be due to the prevailing economic circumstances, but it is also certainly related to her drinking. She has been quite drunk at work on occasion and is struggling to control the business effectively. She sees drinking as a requirement of her work, both in the workplace and in socialising and networking and has recently stopped using her car when she attends these events.

She describes her drinking as having increased since soon after the birth of her son and having escalated around the time of her separation, though her then-partner was unhappy about her level of drinking. She complains of feeling tired and of memory loss after drinking at work.

they both drink too much, resulting in quite different consequences.

2. Is change equally feasible for both individuals? This seems unlikely on the basis of the resources that are available to Janice. She has a business and income, a supportive family (and children) who have expressed concern and may be reasonably intact psychologically. In a general sense, this defines her *social/recovery capital*. The opposing side to this is that the supports available to her could be diminished or lost by continued drinking, thus defining her "current concerns" and commitment to change.

3. In contrast, John's deprived background and the severity of his current life situation mean that he has very little in the way of recovery capital, other than a desire to work allied to periods of sobriety at different points in his life. He appears to have little to lose by comparison. This reflects the tendency for higher levels of social/recovery capital among middle-class problem drinkers as a predictor of recovery.

4. In both cases, attention should be paid to the resources or recovery capital, which they both possess, as well as the elements that need to be mobilised in order to support recovery. An element of recovery that is potentially predictive is that of self-efficacy (i.e. the extent to which an individual believes that they are capable of change).

5. Janice could be a "self-changer", enlisting support from those around her to sustain change. Alternatively, she could be a treatment seeker; however, her family and business commitments would suggest that she be offered help in the context of community-based services or out-patient care and support.

6. Recovery for John would look quite different given his previous life experiences and supports. His unstable situation suggests that he is unlikely to be a successful "self-changer". Should he decide to opt for more formal help, he would commonly be involved in a residential care setting for those with alcohol problems, frequently described as "rehabilitation", where a wide range of social supports and opportunities would be available (e.g. individual and group intervention for alcohol dependence, employability, and independent living skills). Such services would commonly support attendance at 12-step meetings (AA) and, in some instances, offer supported accommodation in the medium term to assist in a return to independent living within the community. He is most likely to be offered support for abstinence.

7. Recovery for Janice could involve the retention of her business and family, and the support and reinforcement that all these things offer. She may continue to consume alcohol, or may abstain, either way seeking support in

that decision and engaging in non-drinking social activities.

8. Both may benefit from social support for harm-free drinking or abstinence. In the long term, the recovery needs for both individuals are likely to be very different. In both cases, their needs and effective supports are likely to change over time, reflecting other developments in their lives.

9. With regard to personal identity, it is quite likely that they would have different ideas about whether they would consider or describe themselves as former problem drinkers. The proposed recovery trajectory for John may make it difficult for him to divest himself of the "recovering alcoholic" label. This would not be the case for Janice, given the potential for her to recover without a lengthy recovery trajectory constructed for her by mutual self-help groups and rehabilitation services.

Specialist treatment: Part of recovery for some

Treatment seekers

Treatment seekers are a diverse group, and differences between them and self-changers are neither dramatic nor consistent (Di Clemente, 2006). They are commonly people who have experienced prolonged problems and have been unsuccessful at self-change and feel the need, or are motivated by others, to seek help outside of their own social network.

It is clear that for severely dependent and chronic drinkers, greater complications and additional problems (difficulties with relationships, health, employment, alcohol-related offences and control over drinking) can make recovery more difficult and influence a decision to seek help. Treatment seekers tend to have lower levels of personal and social capital and greater levels of vulnerability (Raistrick et al., 2006; Best et al., 2010). It is not uncommon to find individuals in specialist alcohol services who have lost a great deal in life due to their drinking and who consequently have few resources and opportunities available to them. The absence of these resources predicts poor treatment or recovery outcomes and, in turn, may increase dependence on treatment services.

A brief history of treatment research

In the UK, 100 married male alcoholics were randomly assigned to either a comprehensive 3-hour assessment (including goal setting for abstinence) or the optimum NHS treatment for alcohol dependence, which involves access to in-patient facilities, psychiatrists, and social workers. At follow-up 12 and 24 months later, the outcomes for drinking for both groups were identical. This finding confirmed that more treatment did not necessarily result in better outcomes. While the amount of treatment offered made no difference, client characteristics (marital cohesion, self-esteem, and job status), which are synonymous with recovery capital, were predictive of success or failure (Orford and Edwards, 1977). This body of research, in addition to subsequent replications, had a profound effect on the nature of specialist treatment for alcohol problems and prompted a move to shorter duration in-patient services and a move towards community-based services.

From the mid-1970s to the mid-1990s, the research literature on treatment effectiveness concluded that structured treatments for alcohol-related problems produced superior results, in most cases, when compared to "control" groups. In other words, treatment as it was worked better than nothing. However, research also demonstrated the absence of a superior intervention. Subsequently, three themes emerged, which have formed the basis of treatment research: first, client-treatment matching studies where treatment effectiveness may be enhanced by matching the treatment type to client characteristics; second, investigation of the impact of combined pharmacological and psychosocial interventions; and third, the investigation of common processes of change inherent in all psychosocial interventions, based on similarity of treatment outcomes.

Treatment matching

Project MATCH (Matching Alcoholism Treatment and Client Heterogeneity),

conducted in the USA, and UKATT (United Kingdom Alcohol Treatment Trial, 2008) are the most important treatment-matching studies. In MATCH, three interventions were compared (see Box 3.4) and delivered in a manual format. The aim of the study was to identify the best outcome produced by a combination of client characteristics and the method of intervention. The goal in all three interventions was abstinence.

The findings of Project MATCH surprised the alcohol-treatment research field, as the matching of client characteristics to interventions was not supported and drinking outcomes were similar irrespective of intervention or client characteristics (Babor and

---

Box 3.4 Project MATCH interventions

(1) Cognitive–Behavioural Therapy (CBT): a coping skills intervention, based on social learning theory, delivered in 12 sessions over 12 weeks.
(2) Twelve-Step Facilitation (TSF): designed to increase access and AA attendance. Delivered in 12 sessions over 12 weeks (see Box 3.2).
(3) Motivational Enhancement Therapy (MET): based on cognitive and motivational psychology and delivered in 4 sessions over a 12-week period.

Del Boca, 2003). The UKATT (2008) sought to explore the implications of Project MATCH for UK treatment services (Raistrick et al., 2006). This study compared the established effectiveness of an extended brief intervention, Motivational Enhancement Therapy (MET), with Social Behaviour Network Therapy (SBNT), which was designed for the trial. Matching hypotheses were identical in both UKATT and MATCH. MET and SBNT showed equivalent outcomes and the UKATT research team concluded that client-treatment matching is unlikely to result in substantial improvement in the effectiveness of treatment for alcohol problems (UKATT, 2008).

The implications of matching studies are that despite significant theoretical differences between the interventions studied in MATCH and UKATT, there appear to be few differences in treatment outcomes as measured by abstinence or levels of alcohol consumption, therefore confirming that there are many effective interventions. Both MATCH and UKATT underline the importance of providing well-structured and "manual" interventions that are delivered by well-trained staff. However, the issue of matching services to client characteristics does not rest there. There are other ways in which treatment seekers are matched to services. In the absence of treatment matching to client characteristics, UKATT (2008) reinforces the importance of clinical/professional judgement in relation to creating treatment interventions that

meet the needs of the service users, including the need for ongoing support after treatment (SMACAP, 2011). In service delivery settings, whether health or social care, the theme of clinical or professional judgement based on an assessment of individual need is fundamental to matching client needs to the interventions and services required. This is consistent with person-centred care and supports the importance of the client–therapist alliance.

Pharmacological interventions

There are three pharmacological approaches that are relevant to treatment for alcohol dependence: detoxification for safe withdrawal, nutritional supplementation, and relapse prevention. In this section, evidence for the use of pharmacological interventions will be described, and combined psychosocial and pharmacological interventions will be evaluated.

Detoxification

Many dependent drinkers stop by themselves without the aid of medication, although it is not without risks, including uncomfortable withdrawal symptoms. Those in contact with medical services and who seek specialist treatment for an alcohol problem may be offered detoxification medication, with an emphasis on safety. Detoxification is usually achieved rapidly, commonly in 5–10 days, during which withdrawal symptoms (notably sweats, nausea, tremor) and serious medical complications (such as withdrawal seizures and dementia tremens) are minimised. The drug of choice for detoxification is chlordiazepoxide (Librium). A Librium prescription is restricted to the withdrawal period, as further use tends to increase tolerance and dependence as well as interact with alcohol (NICE, 2010a,b). The achievement of detoxification is a common starting point for treatment and is viewed as required to prevent relapse (Slattery et al., 2003). The use of benzodiazepines revolutionised the treatment of alcohol withdrawal and has reduced the risk of death associated with detoxification (O'Malley and Kosten, 2006).

Nutritional supplements

Thiamine deficiency is a feature of heavy drinking, where poor diet is a feature. Wernicke's encephalopathy is a serious consequence of thiamine deficiency, with symptoms including confusion, ophthalmoplegia and ataxia; this condition can be treated by thiamine booster. Failure to spot and treat Wernicke's will result in Korsakoff's syndrome, which includes serious alcohol-related brain damage and enduring memory impairment.

Relapse prevention

Medication must be consumed if it is to have any effect; consequently, studies about the effectiveness of medications used to treat alcohol dependence usually have a substantial amount of psychosocial

support in order to enhance drug compliance.

Disulfiram is a sensitising medication that produces a negative reaction to alcohol by interfering with liver enzymes in the breakdown of acetaldehyde when it is consumed prior to drinking alcohol. When the individual taking disulfiram consumes alcohol, the drug produces symptoms such as headache, vomiting, nausea, flushing and tachycardia. Thus, the expected positive outcomes from drinking are changed to negative outcomes. The individual's knowledge of the reaction and their commitment to taking the medication are crucial, and, over time, the negative associations to consuming alcohol may result in stable abstinence. Administration of disulfiram is commonly supervised, either by a relative or programme staff (O'Malley and Kosten, 2006). Disulfiram's purpose is to maintain abstinence and thereby prevent relapse. Disulfiram is recommended by the Health Technology Board, Scotland (HTBS), National Treatment Agency (NTA) and the National Institute for Clinical Excellence (NICE).

Acamprosate may reduce the physiological and psychological distress and cravings that result from alcohol withdrawal and are cued by environmental stimuli. A meta-analysis concluded that abstinence rates at 6 months were significantly higher in the acamprosate-treated group compared to a control group (O'Malley and Kosten, 2006). Acamprosate is recommended by HTBS, NTA, and NICE.

Naltrexone is an opioid antagonist, which blocks the effects of opioid drugs such as heroin or methadone at the receptor sites in the central nervous system. It is commonly used to reverse opioid overdose and may partially block the pleasurable effects of alcohol, thereby reducing the risk of relapse. Naltrexone has been investigated in 15 studies involving 2300 alcohol-dependent individuals, and the majority of the studies demonstrate improved outcomes over placebo treatment (O'Malley and Kosten, 2006). Naltrexone is recommended by Raistrick et al. (2006) and NICE (2010a,b).

In a meta-analysis, researchers concluded that acamprosate was slightly more effective in supporting abstinence while naltrexone was slightly more effective in reducing cravings and heavy drinking (Maisel et al., 2013).

Combining pharmacological and cognitive–behavioural interventions

Few studies have investigated the combined effects of psychosocial interventions and medication. Project COMBINE (Anton et al., 2006) tested the impact of naltrexone and acamprosate in a variety of combinations with a package of cognitive–behavioural interventions (including motivational interviewing, coping skills, community support, and TSF) described as combined behavioural intervention (CBI). Both drugs showed minor benefits over control groups when combined with CBI. Naltrexone was best suited to individuals who had lapsed because it inhibits heavy drinking, while acamprosate appeared best suited to those concerned about possible relapse (Anton et al., 2006; Raistrick et al., 2006; NICE, 2011).

!	Thinking Point
What is the importance of medication in a CBI?	

Treatment-outcome similarity

Treatment-outcome comparison studies produced similar results. There are a number of factors that may contribute to similarity of outcomes among the differing treatments. Some of these influences are a function of the research design and procedures, while others are aspects of the treatment setting and the client–therapist therapeutic alliance.

Problem drinkers who have mental health, homelessness, or poly-drug use issues are often excluded from treatment-outcome research, as these characteristics make it more difficult to follow up with these individuals. The exclusion of the more difficult or troubled individuals makes the remaining subjects more homogenous and limits the generalisability of findings to less vulnerable service users.

The selection process for treatment-outcome studies tends to be rigorous and may involve several hours of assessment for study inclusion, prior to administration of the intervention being tested. Assessment for Project MATCH took more than 5 hours, while by comparison MET in both MATCH and UKATT lasted no more than 4 hours. It is feasible that a comprehensive assessment for the purpose of inclusion, or exclusion, from a research project may equate to a treatment intervention in terms of outcome. Furthermore, such assessment will be given to all subjects, irrespective of their inclusion in the treatment or control groups, and this assessment may obscure measurable differences among the interventions being tested and control conditions.

Despite theoretical differences, there are potent common ingredients in the treatment interventions tested in MATCH and UKATT, which may explain the similarities in outcomes. For example, Cognitive Behavioural Therapy (CBT), which focuses on coping skill development, will also support motivation to change and enhance self-belief, both of which are substantial elements of Motivational Enhancement Therapy. Similarly TSF, as evidenced by AA attendance, will support motivation, provide direct coping advice ("one day at a time"), and provide a non-drinking social environment. Nevertheless, the "equal outcome" phenomenon has been a feature of general psychotherapy outcome research for a variety of psychotherapeutic interventions (Berglund, 2005). The idea of common processes across all treatments, based on identical outcomes,

also has strong support. A contrary perspective is proposed by Orford (2008), who concludes "that apparently contrasting treatments are, in most respects, not different at all". Psychotherapeutic treatment-outcome research concludes that active ingredients are attributed to "general" factors (Berglund, 2005; Orford, 2008). This is consistent with a change and recovery perspective, where a wide range of life factors have primacy, in influencing both change and its maintenance, over specialist treatment interventions.

Therapist characteristics and therapeutic alliance

Treatment trials, by definition, attempt to control therapist variables or characteristics by training therapists to a consistent level and commonly using treatment manuals as a means to demonstrate the impact of the treatment technique alone. A key feature of competent practitioners is their ability to create a therapeutic alliance with the service user. Therapist characteristics (empathy, supportiveness, goal orientation and promotion of self-determination) and the therapeutic alliance are important and commonly reported by treatment subjects at follow-up, more so than the particular intervention technique tested (Saunders and Kershaw, 1979; Orford, 2008). The understanding of client needs and the ability to be flexible and effectively deviate from a prescribed treatment intervention, in some respects, mirrors the therapeutic alliance associated with positive treatment outcomes. Therapist characteristics are an important ingredient in treatment delivery and may account for up to 50% of outcomes. "A half century of psychotherapy research has demonstrated that the most robust predictor of treatment success is the quality of the therapeutic alliance" (Nilsen, 2010). There is no evidence to suggest that these positive therapist characteristics are more common among "recovering alcoholics"; consequently, the belief that "only an alcoholic can help an alcoholic" is not supported.

These factors contribute to what is perceived by service users as a credible treatment or service. In addition, these factors make service users feel as if someone is paying attention to them and give service users a sense of hope.

What should specialist treatment look like?

Treatment-outcome research reviews

A number of reviews of treatment-outcome research were conducted in the early 21st century, all with the aim of summarising international evidence about the effectiveness of treatment interventions for moderate to severe alcohol dependence. Two such research reviews were conducted in the UK.

The *Health Technology Board for Scotland* (HTBS) (Slattery et al., 2003) conducted a systematic review of the scientific treatment literature, including "evidence from experts and professional groups, manufacturers and other interested parties". The review sought to identify which treatments (psychosocial and pharmacological) would yield the maximum maintenance of recovery amongst those dependent on alcohol, who had been detoxified and were newly abstinent, and were therefore ready to engage with *relapse prevention*-focused interventions. The following interventions were recommended: behavioural self-control training, MET, marital/family therapy, coping/social skills training plus access to voluntary organisations and 12-step groups, and pharmacological interventions (see above).

The *National Treatment Agency* (England and Wales) (NTA) review (Raistrick et al., 2006) provides a perspective on evidence-informed treatments, taking into account both the drinking culture and service structures in the UK. The NTA review (Raistrick et al., 2006) has cast its net wide in its recommendations for evidence-based interventions, resulting in considerable choice of psychosocial interventions, which is reflected in clinical guidelines (NICE, 2011) (Box 3.5).

In light of the above, clarity is required in order to specify the functions and processes that constitute specialist treatment for harmful drinking and dependence. Services for problem drinkers should be person-centred, reflecting a trusting relationship that

---

Box 3.5 NICE (2011) clinical guidance: Summary of key priorities

Clinical Guidance 115 was designed to provide clear guidance on the details of identification and treatment of alcohol dependence and, by implication, recovery.

Identification and assessment in all settings. Staff working in services provided and funded by the NHS who care for people who potentially misuse alcohol should be able to identify harmful drinking and alcohol dependence.

Assessment in specialist alcohol services. Comprehensive assessment for all adults who score more than 15 on the Alcohol Use Disorders Identification Test (AUDIT) covering the following areas:

alcohol consumption, including:
drinking history and recent pattern of drinking; other drug use; and, if possible, additional information from a family member or carer

(1) degree of dependence, which can be measured by the Severity of Alcohol Dependence Questionnaire (SADQ) or Leeds Dependence Questionnaire (LDQ)

- alcohol-related problems
- physical health problems
- psychological problems
- social problems (including family, employment, and criminal justice matters)

(2) cognitive function (Mini-Mental State Examination)
(3) risk to self and others
(4) readiness and belief in ability to change
(5) recovery capital

---

is supportive, empathic, and non-judgemental. Account should be taken of the stigma and discrimination that may be part of the experience of having an alcohol problem. A focus on individual needs and preferences thus will enable treatment providers to make informed decisions (NICE, 2011; SMACAP, 2011). These elements form the "therapeutic alliance".

Specialist treatments for severe alcohol problems are predominantly psychological and environmental in nature, based on talking therapies plus the appropriate use of pharmacological interventions as an adjunct, particularly in relation to moderate to severe dependence (see section on "Mutual self-help").

General principles for all interventions

Offer interventions to promote abstinence and prevent relapse as part of an intensive structured, community-based intervention for people with moderate to severe alcohol dependence, with limited social support, or complex physical or psychiatric comorbidities, or those who have not responded to initial community-based interventions.

All interventions (psychological and pharmacological) should be delivered by appropriately trained and competent staff. Psychological interventions should be based on evidence-based treatment manuals.

The individuals being treated should be involved in reviewing the effectiveness of their treatment plans. A recovery perspective will allow the individual to plan for aftercare support (beyond the treatment intervention).

Interventions for harmful drinking and mild alcohol dependence: offer psychological intervention.

Assessment for assisted alcohol withdrawal: for those who drink over 15 units of alcohol per day and/or who score 20 or more on the Alcohol Use Disorders Identification Test (AUDIT), consider offering assessment for community-based assisted withdrawal or management in specialist alcohol services if there are safety concerns.

Interventions for moderate and severe alcohol dependence: after successful withdrawal, consider offering

acamprosate or oral naltrexone in combination with an individual psychological intervention.

Assessment and interventions for children and young people who misuse alcohol: for children and young people 10–17 years old who misuse alcohol, offer individual cognitive–behavioural therapy and family therapies for those with significant comorbidities and/or limited social support.

Interventions for conditions comorbid with alcohol misuse: for people who have comorbid depression or anxiety disorders, the alcohol problem should be dealt with as a priority; this may lead to improvement in the depression and anxiety. If these symptoms persist after 3–4 weeks of abstinence from alcohol, consider referral.

Thinking Point
(1) What role does the therapeutic alliance play in recovery?
(2) What are the optimum therapist characteristics?

Summary Points
1. In the absence of treatment, change is seldom spontaneous, natural or unaided. Natural recovery and treatment are intertwined. The common feature is change, a process which underlies all recovery.
2. Generally higher socio-economic status and social stability are predictive of greater recovery from alcohol dependence.

Continued

3. Recovery takes a long-term view of change, and the development of innovative means of support and enhancement of social capital is important.

4. Treatment has its place in the recovery journey for some, and its effectiveness has been demonstrated.

5. Given the similarities in health care provisions across the UK, the HTBS and NTA review recommendations are of particular importance.

6. The weight of evidence lies with the cognitive–behavioural family of interventions. However, this may obscure the potential use of less well-researched interventions.

7. The importance of change processes, irrespective of treatment techniques, has led to calls for further investigation of change processes.

8. Professional and clinical judgements should reflect a person-centred, recovery-focused approach, ensuring that individual needs are identified and met.

9. Intervention techniques delivered by highly trained, competent, and committed staff, in well-organised and supportive service settings where therapist skills and therapeutic alliances are maximised, is central to optimal treatment outcomes.

10. Mutual self-help groups, particularly 12-step organisations, function as an alternative to treatment and as post-treatment support for recovery.

11. Even with the most effective current treatment (for example, cognitive–behavioural therapies and social network and environment-based therapies), the effects are modest at best and the treatments are not effective for everyone.

12. People move in and out of different drinking behaviours and change is best conceptualised as a process, which may or may not be assisted by treatment. There are many social influences that have greater effectiveness than treatment.

Web pages and resources

http://guidance.nice.org.uk/CG115
  National Institute for Clinical Excellence Alcohol Guidance
http://www.alcoholics-anonymous.org.uk/
  Alcoholics Anonymous
https://www.drinkaware.co.uk/make-a-change
  Drinkaware
http://scotland.gov.uk/Publications/2011/03/18085806/0
  Practice-oriented document offering a broader perspective than clinical guidance on alcohol recovery and supportive interventions. Relevant to all service settings.

Further reading

Raistrick, D., Heather, N., Godfrey, C., 2006. Review of the Effectiveness of Treatment for Alcohol Problems. National Treatment Agency for Substance Misuse. NHS.
An excellent review of alcohol treatment in the UK, providing a flexible perspective on choice of intervention.

Scottish Ministerial Advisory Committee on Alcohol Problems, 2011. Quality Alcohol Treatment SMACAP Scottish Government, Edinburgh.
Encapsulates the development of a recovery perspective in the development of quality services for problem drinkers.

4 Family and workplace

This chapter describes the impact of alcohol on the family and the workplace. In it, we examine the role of the family in the socialisation of young drinkers, the impact of harmful drinking on the family (including domestic violence and child welfare), and a brief outline of evidence-based interventions that involve the family in the resolution of problem drinking. We consider the impact of alcohol on the workplace, the potential of workplace policies to reduce drinking, and the challenge of engaging employers in the resolution of work-based alcohol issues.

The role of the family in socialising young drinkers

Children are socialised into drinking cultures and have a concept of alcohol long before they actually consume it. One research study demonstrates that, at the age of four, many children can distinguish between alcohol and other drinks bottles, and, at the age of six, on seeing a film of a person who is staggering, many children will conclude that the person is drunk rather than ill. Many parents give young children sips of diluted alcoholic drinks in the belief that the home is the best place to learn about alcohol; this belief is based on their own experiences of alcohol rather than health messages. Despite this, parents are more likely to suggest that the mid-teens is the best age to introduce young people to alcohol (Valentine et al., 2010).

The family is the main source of influence on younger children, and a dynamic and complex series of parent–child interactions regarding alcohol shape the emergent drinking behaviour. As in many other matters, the family unit ensures the transfer of culturally approved, though sometimes risky, attitudes and behaviours regarding alcohol (Eadie et al., 2010). As the young person moves into adolescence, peer groups and media become greater influences. Drinking confers social standing and peer acceptance, making the struggle to cope with initially unpleasant-tasting drinks worthwhile. Because of peer acceptance, young people were more likely to admit to drinking recently and admit to the amounts of alcohol they consumed if they believed that most of their friends consumed alcohol (Eadie et al., 2010).

Some studies describe an implicit contract between parents and children, where the parents know about the young person's drinking but have not necessarily seen the young person intoxicated (Percy et al., 2010). One strategy adopted by young people is to drink to excess earlier in the evening and return home more sober; this is an aspect of binge drinking (see Chapter 1 for more information on binge drinking). Young people in the UK tend to drink to get drunk, despite health messages emphasising moderation. Drinking and getting drunk is therefore a skill, strongly reinforced by peer culture, the observation of elders, and the influence of product promotions. Risky drinking in young people conforms to cultural norms and forms part of a rite of passage of the adolescent towards adulthood. Young people do not have a drinking culture that is discrete and unconnected to the broader adult drinking culture. Indeed, most adults would describe their youthful drinking as risky and similar to that of young people.

Family relationships may protect against alcohol problems; however, the socialisation process may not always go as we might hope. Some aspects of family life seem to be associated with alcohol problems in young people and later in life. Problem drinking seems to run in families and is associated with a myriad of influences. Family instability and excessive drinking itself in a parent, or parents, may result in more extreme attitudes and behaviour in the younger person, either in favour of excessive drinking or abstinence (Sondhi and Turner, 2011). In an Australian study, more frequent partner change by parents, coupled with lower levels of control over younger children was a strong predictor of adolescents drinking. Problem drinking in adolescents may be influenced by peer networks, parental attempts to manage adolescent behaviour, and long standing negative parent–child relationships (Alati et al., 2010). Abused or maltreated children are at increased risk of developing poorer behavioural, educational and mental health outcomes, including substance use problems later in life (Galvani, 2010; Laslett et al., 2012). About two-thirds of people seeking specialist treatment report having a parent with an alcohol problem (Scottish Executive, 2003). Many of these themes are incorporated into alcohol education targeting young people and their families. (See Chapter 5 for more information about public health alcohol interventions.)

The impact of the problem drinker on the family

In separate surveys in New Zealand and Australia, a relationship was found between reduced quality of life, poor health and contact with heavy drinkers. In both studies, about 30% of respondents reported having at least one heavy drinker in their life, and 25% indicated that the heavy drinker lived in their household. Negative consequences associated with the drinker were consistently reported, with 11% affected 'a lot'. The harms reported ranged from noise and fear to physical abuse, sexual coercion and social isolation (Casswell et al., 2011; Laslett et al., 2011).

The impact on those living with a harmful/dependent drinker is further demonstrated in a US study (Ray et al., 2009), where family members of people suffering from chronic conditions (diabetes and asthma) were compared to the families of dependent drinkers. The latter suffered more trauma, depression and alcohol and drug problems, resulting in greater use of, and costs to, health services. Separation from a male problem drinker reduces the likelihood of alcohol-related problems among female partners (Smith et al., 2012).

The implication is that harmful and dependent drinkers may have a negative impact on those around them. The issue is further complicated depending on family structure; the impacts may also be quite different, depending on which family member is the problem drinker. These findings are important as they raise the issue of the unmeasured impact and costs of alcohol on families in the community as opposed to the families of those who use specialist alcohol treatment services.

Alcohol-related domestic abuse and violence

Domestic abuse covers a range of negative experiences: emotional, sexual, physical, financial and psychological abuse. Alcohol is often present and contributes to domestic violence, but it is neither a necessary nor a sufficient cause. Men are most commonly the perpetrators, and women (and children) the victims. Intoxication neither explains nor excuses abuse or violence though it is often used as an excuse by perpetrators. Similarly, some victims blame the alcohol rather than the perpetrator.

In the UK, more than 60% of cases of domestic violence involve alcohol (Home Office, 2004). English probation services records show that the majority of domestic violence offenders (62%) had consumed alcohol, and almost half the sample (48%) were alcohol dependent (Gilchrist et al., 2003). In domestic violence incidents reported to Northumbria police, the perpetrators' use of alcohol, particularly heavy drinking, resulted in more serious injuries to their partners. Men's violence was more severe than that of women and commonly involved alcohol (Hester, 2009).

Women who experience domestic abuse are up to 15 times more likely to misuse alcohol than women in the general population (Alcohol Concern, 2010a,b). They also have a lower rate of completion of specialist treatment programmes compared to non-abused women who are problem drinkers. Women in abusive relationships commonly report drinking and drug use as a coping mechanism; consequently, current abuse would undermine the impact of treatment for alcohol dependence.

Child welfare

Alcohol misuse by a parent can seriously disrupt parenting and child care and creates significant problems for child care systems (Harbin and Murphy, 2000) (Box 4.1).

Parents' drinking does not necessarily result in harm to children; however, for some it does. A study of calls to Childline Scotland explored how children express their concerns about their parents' drinking, the effect it has on their lives, and how they coped (Wales and Gillan, 2009). Children reported severe emotional distress, physical abuse and violence, and a general lack of care and

protection. Most children stated that violence (ranging from being slapped to being punched and kicked) happened when the parent was drunk or had been drinking. The importance of this type of finding is that it is based on self-reports from a community population as opposed to a child welfare population or the children of those in treatment for alcohol dependence. The wider literature on parental alcohol and drug use demonstrates a close link between problem substance use and child neglect or maltreatment, including violence.

An Australian study of 29,455 children found an association between alcohol or drug problems and recurrent child maltreatment and indicated that almost 25% of the children identified experienced a second incident of maltreatment within a 5-year period. Where the carer was identified as having

---

Box 4.1 Some indicators of the impact of alcohol on children in the UK

- It is estimated that 2.6 million children in the UK live with parents who drink hazardously; 705,000 children live with dependent drinkers; 65,000 Scottish children live in a household where a parent's drinking is problematic.
- More than 100 children a week call Childline about a parent's drinking or drug use.
- 62% of children subject to care proceedings in the London boroughs have parents who misuse substances.
- 25–33% of known cases of child abuse are associated with alcohol.
- 57% of case reviews of serious abuse involve parental substance misuse.
- 78% of young offenders who misuse alcohol have a history of parental alcohol abuse or domestic abuse.

Sources: Alcohol Concern (2010b) (http://www.alcoholconcern.org.uk/assets/files/ Publications/Swept%20under%20the%20carpet.pdf; accessed 14 February 2013) and Scottish Government (2008a,b)).

an alcohol problem, the children were significantly more likely to experience multiple incidents. Furthermore, the caregiver who was a problem drinker was not necessarily the perpetrator of the violence, but the enduring nature of an alcohol problem in a parent may leave children vulnerable (Laslett et al., 2012). In an investigation of 50 families with 95 children who were on the Child Protection Register in inner London, researchers concluded that substance use had a significant negative impact on children in 52% of cases; the primary problem substances were alcohol (24%) and heroin (16%) (Forrester, 2000).

These findings are important in terms of child welfare procedures in the UK, where all agencies in contact with children and their families have a responsibility to act if they become worried about a child's welfare or a parent's ability to care for the child safely and adequately. The welfare of the child is the paramount consideration. If a child is at risk of harm, this risk must override concerns about the parent's wishes or welfare (Scottish Executive, 2003). This ethos underpins child welfare and protection across the UK (The Advisory Council on the Misuse of Drugs (ACMD), 2007; Scottish Government, 2010).

Some parents are faced with a very difficult dilemma regarding their substance use and their role as a parent. In one study, women who were severely dependent upon alcohol felt that if they sought treatment this might prevent authorities from removing their children from their homes and placing the children into care. At the same time, they were afraid that requesting treatment might increase the risk of their children being taken from them (Powis et al., 2000). These beliefs and fears are strongly held among families where alcohol is a problem, despite the significant development of family- and child-focused services in recent years and increased awareness of family and child welfare issues in specialist addiction services. Child welfare practitioners have a difficult task: to recognise and act upon the needs of the child in the face of harmful drinking.

> **! Thinking Point**
>
> How can children be made safer and more resilient in families affected by harmful drinking?

Family-focused interventions and recovery

The family is an important source of support and reinforcement for behaviour change, thus mediating the impact of specialist treatment. There is long-standing evidence that the nature and quality of marital and family relationships has a significant impact on treatment outcomes and recovery, for better or worse, and that the social network is important in sustaining change or preventing relapse (Orford and Edwards, 1977; McCready, 2006; The United Kingdom Alcohol Treatment Trial (UKATT), 2008). Most family-focused interventions attempt to alter sources of reinforcement in the client's environment in order to diminish substance use (Meyers and Miller, 2001).

Specialist treatment for alcohol dependence has significant benefits for the recovering drinker's family. Family members report improved mental health, reduced stress, an increase in quality of life, and reduced expenditure and time spent caring for the individual 1 year after detoxification for alcohol dependence. These are important but often neglected benefits of treatment (Salize et al., 2013).

Four types of family-focused intervention

(1) Interventions which seek to meet the needs of family members

Al-Anon is based on 12-step principles, like Alcoholics Anonymous (see Chapter 3), and espouses the view that as alcoholism is a disease, the partner who attends Al-Anon can only change themselves, not the drinker. It is without doubt the best-known support organisation for the partners and friends of problem drinkers. Studies evaluating the impact of interventions that target the concerned significant other

(CSO) consistently report that those who engage with Al-Anon, which is designed to enhance coping skills, experience marked reductions in what were high levels of stress and mental ill health. Al-Anon's focus on the needs of the drinker's family members means it is less effective in encouraging treatment of the problem drinker (Roozen et al., 2010).

http://www.al-anonuk.org.uk/about/is-al-anon-for-you.html

5-Step was tested on people affected by the alcohol or drug use of a close family member in the Midlands and South West England. Relatives (143) were randomly allocated to either a full or brief intervention. The full intervention consisted of up to five sessions (5-Step), using a structured manual focusing on substance use, stress coping, and support; the family member was given a self-help version of the intervention manual. The brief intervention consisted of one session, during which the content of the self-help manual was explained and the family member was encouraged to make use of the manual. There was no difference in stress and coping measures between the two groups when followed up after 3 months; thus, the self-help manual was as effective as several face-to-face contacts between professionals and family members (Copello et al., 2009a,b).

The five steps are:

1. Listen non-judgementally
2. Provide information
3. Discuss ways of responding
4. Explore sources of support
5. Arrange further help if needed

(2) Interventions designed to meet the needs of family members and encourage the drinker to access treatment

This group of interventions is often described as unilateral because the decision to seek help is made by family members irrespective of the problem drinkers' wishes.

Community Reinforcement and Family Training (*CRAFT*) has shown psychosocial and health improvements equivalent to Al-Anon (Roozen et al., 2010). Similarly, studies of treatment outcomes for alcohol dependence report a reduction in concerned significant others' stress levels when problem drinking is reduced or ceases (Copello and Orford, 2002; Orford et al., 2005). However, CRAFT was found to be superior in engaging treatment-resistant individuals compared to traditional programmes, demonstrating three times more patient engagement than Al-Anon. CRAFT encouraged two-thirds of treatment-resistant individuals to attend four to six CRAFT sessions (Myers et al., 2001).

CRAFT consists of:

1. Developing a trusting relationship
2. Preparing the CSO to recognise and respond to the potential for domestic violence, including seeking safety
3. Functional analysis for (a) triggers for drinking and (b) triggers for non-drinking
4. Improving communications
5. Training the CSO to use positive reinforcement and negative consequences
6. Stress reduction
7. Assisting the CSO to introduce the topic of treatment and lay groundwork for service access (Myers et al., 2001)

Bottled up is a membership Web site designed to support relatives and friends of problem drinkers. It is distinct from Al-Anon, using evidence based on principles of learning theory. Success is achieved by rewarding improvements in behaviour and working towards change and treatment (McMahon and Lewis, 2010; Bottled up: http://bottled-up.memberlodge.com (accessed 1 July 2013).

(3) Interventions for the family/social network to support change in the problem drinker

Social Behaviour and Network Therapy (SBNT) is based on the principle that social behaviour, interaction and network support for behaviour play important roles in the resolution of alcohol and addiction problems. SBNT is as effective as Motivational

Enhancement Therapy in reducing alcohol consumption (UKATT, 2008). SBNT focuses on the person with a drinking problem and proceeds to identify family members and friends who support this person's efforts to change; SBNT engages these family members and friends in the treatment process as much as possible. The aim is to assist clients to develop social networks that support change. SBNT consists of the following core elements (Copello et al., 2009a,b):

1. Identify social network membership
2. Enhance communication
3. Explore coping
4. Enhance social support
5. Network-based relapse prevention
6. Plus electives on alcohol information, employment, developing support, and increasing pleasant and joint activities

(4) Integrated programmes for mothers

These programmes target women and have a strong child welfare element; these programmes also include a wide range of interventions, such as individual addiction treatment, maternal mental health services, prenatal education, medical and nutrition services, trauma treatment, life skills training, education and employment assistance, parenting education and counselling, child care, children's services, follow-up and aftercare.

From a systematic review of these programmes, it was suggested that compared to addiction treatment alone, integrated programmes lead to small additional improvements in parenting associated with enhanced attachment-based parenting. In residential settings, children remain with their parent.

Despite the small effect, the impact on the financial and human burden in this vulnerable population could be significant. There could be a reduction in the need for child care and protection services (including foster care), the need for psychiatric admissions, and offending (Niccols et al., 2012).

There are similarities in the array of interventions outlined above. The development of non-judgemental therapeutic relationships is central to all approaches. Significant attention is paid to the family network in terms of the harm attributable to drinking and the potential for the family to support change in the drinker. A crucial by-product of this approach, as opposed to individualised intervention, is the attention that can be paid to domestic abuse, including children's welfare, and the individual needs of family members. Family-focused interventions, which target the whole family or family members but have the secondary objective of engaging the reluctant drinker in treatment, seek to alter and enhance familial relationships and support, and, consequently, diminish the reinforcement of drinking.

Alcohol and the workplace

Workplaces vary greatly in their purpose (commercial, manufacturing or public service), and the make-up of the workforce is also varied in terms of gender, age, social background and ethnicity. Workplace characteristics may also contribute to employee alcohol consumption. Work settings, or types of employment, are affected by alcohol-related issues in different ways, whether relating to accidents, sickness and absence, or matters of conduct.

Impact of alcohol on employers and employees

Harmful alcohol use and heavy episodic drinking increase the risk for problems in the workplace, including absenteeism, reduced performance and productivity, arriving to work late, leaving work early, higher workforce turnover due to illness, inappropriate behaviour, theft and other crimes, other problems that require disciplinary action, poor coworker relations and low company morale. Conversely, structural factors at the workplace, including high stress and low satisfaction, can increase the risk of alcohol use disorders and alcohol dependence (World Health Organisation (WHO), 2009). Box 4.2 summarises the impact of alcohol on UK workplaces.

Box 4.2 The impact of alcohol in the workplace in the UK

- An estimated £6.4 billion annual loss to UK commerce is caused by alcohol.
- Around 200,000 people go to work every day with a hangover.
- An estimated 17 million sick days are taken each year in the UK because of alcohol misuse.
- Sickness absence days in England and Wales increased by over 600,000 per year following the liberalisation of opening hours in 2005.
- Men who drink more than 14 units of alcohol a week are 20% more likely to be absent from work because of injury.
- Internal/company influences on alcohol abuse in the workplace include stress, workload, and latitude of decision making.

Sources: Prime Minister's Strategy Office (2004), Green and Paniagua (2013), Alcohol Concern (2013) (http://www.alcoholconcern.org.uk/workplace).

Diverse work settings, diverse impacts

The impact of alcohol in the workplace depends on the nature of the organisation's activity, the existence and implementation of restrictions on alcohol, and the characteristics of the workforce. Consequently, the impact of alcohol may vary considerably between work settings. Two contrasting examples (white-collar workers/civil servants and members of the armed forces) are presented in Box 4.3.

Addressing alcohol-related harm in the workplace

Reducing the negative impact of alcohol on the workplace is one of five priorities in the *EU strategy to support Member States in reducing alcohol-related harm* (Commission of the European Communities, 2006). The European Alcohol and Health Forum (EAHF) concluded that the complexity of addressing alcohol abuse in the workplace and through the workplace requires a broad and interdisciplinary approach that brings together the efforts of employers and other stakeholders. Multistakeholder partnerships are desirable to improve current approaches and introduce greater consistency in implementation (EAHF, 2011).

Wellness at work

The workplace may contribute to stress in employees as a result of excessive demands and workload, lack of control, and poor relationships with colleagues or managers. Stress produces a range of symptoms and negative outcomes for both individuals and organisations. Government agencies in both the UK and the EU are interested in wellness at work programmes that foster high work performance, employee health and profits. Employees' wellbeing is viewed as the employer's responsibility, with the aim being that staff feel valued, productivity is enhanced and employee absences reduced (Hillier et al., 2005). It is within this context that policies on alcohol in the workplace exist and include various approaches ranging from legislation to prevention efforts and interventions implemented by individual employers. However, a common workplace policy on drinking does not exist across the EU, and action is largely left in the hands of individual employers. As a result, workplace interventions are inconsistent and, in many instances, absent (EU, 2011). One-third of UK businesses do not have an alcohol policy, and most have no strategy in place to reduce the economic costs of alcohol consumption (Alcohol Concern, 2013).

Alcohol policies in the workplace

Responses to alcohol, especially policies in the workplace, originate from the United States, where employers have traditionally been a major source of health care provision for employees through health insurance schemes. In contrast, in the UK, the emergence of such policy approaches has been much

---

Box 4.3 Alcohol in diverse work settings

White-collar workers

White-collar workers, including civil servants, represent a diverse population in both public and commercial work settings. A series of focus groups examined the drinking patterns, perceived norms, and views of the effects of drinking on the personal and professional lives of white-collar workers. Drinking was part of workers' everyday routines, and acceptable consumption, including 'excess', was associated with the ability to function rather than the amount consumed. Public health messages about risk and harm, based on alcohol consumption messages (such as safe limits and units of alcohol), appeared to go unheeded (Ling et al., 2012).

In a study of more than 10,000 UK civil servants, alcohol consumption was related to risk of sickness absence caused by injury. Increased risk was noted in moderate levels of consumption. Binge drinking and alcohol dependence were also related to absence caused by injury (HSE, 2002). Alcohol dependence was associated with low levels of decision-making responsibilities and high levels of effort combined with few rewards.

Armed forces

Recruitment for the armed forces is weighted towards groups in the general population that have a high risk of alcohol misuse, namely young, single males and recruits from deprived socio-economic backgrounds.

In the British armed forces, 67% of men and 49% of women were hazardous drinkers; these levels were significantly higher than in the general population (Fear et al., 2007). Around 75% of violent offences amongst soldiers involve alcohol. In those suffering from combat stress, 20% drank hazardously, and 27% were probably dependent on alcohol. Troops returning from an operational theatre were 22% more likely to have an alcohol problem than those not deployed (Ministry of Defence, 2010).

A survey of 1,333 male personnel in the Royal Navy from 12 operational ships found that 92% were hazardous drinkers, 25% drank more than double the recommended weekly safe limit, 48% reported binge drinking at least once a week, and 15% were problem drinkers. The researchers concluded that high levels of drinking are now likely to impact occupational efficiency and that alcohol also has a very positive influence on military culture: units that drink more have better cohesion and higher morale (Ministry of Defence, 2010). Alcohol has been taken more seriously as a disciplinary, health and performance issue by the armed forces. Further concerns have been expressed that heavy drinking is too ingrained in military life and that alcohol problems may become apparent when an individual tries to re-enter civilian life (Alcohol Concern Cymru, 2012).

less evident. While this reflects differing cultural attitudes towards alcohol and sobriety, it also reflects the level of state provision of health care, reducing the need for or likelihood of the employer to take an active role. Consequently, the slow development of alcohol policies in the workplace in the UK may be a direct result of the existing state health care provision.

There is strong support for alcohol, and other health-related policies in the workplace from organisations that have interests in health, health and safety, and industrial relations, such as Alcohol Concern, the International Labour Organisation (ILO), the Trades Union Congress (TUC), the Advisory Conciliation and Arbitration Service (ACAS) and the Office of Fair Trading (OFT), despite a lack of enthusiasm from employers.

There are many sources for model policies. While there is great similarity among all of them, policies should be tailored to the needs of the organisation and its workforce in consultation with relevant parties, including trade unions. The creation and implementation of a workplace policy has the potential to prevent alcohol problems as well as help individual employees manage alcohol problems. In the latter case, workplace policies tend to feature both disciplinary and assistance dimensions. The assistance element of a workplace policy allows disciplinary actions to be suspended while the employee participates in a treatment programme; 80% of employers treat

alcohol issues as a combination of disciplinary and health issues (Chartered Institute of Personnel Development, 2007).

Workplace policies can also provide an opportunity for harm reduction (Box 4.4). In an Australian survey of 300 first-year apprentices (aged 15–22 years), more than 40% reported cannabis and alcohol consumption patterns that placed them at risk of harm. Approximately 19% drank alcohol and 7% reported using cannabis during work-related hours. Workplace availability of alcohol and the existence of workplace policies were associated with consumption patterns. Those employed in workplaces where alcohol was available drank more often than those reporting no alcohol availability at work. Those reporting an alcohol policy at their workplace reported less alcohol use compared to apprentices reporting no policy. Workplace factors, particularly workplace policies, were associated with young employees' alcohol and drug use both at and outside the workplace (Pidd et al., 2006).

Testing employees for alcohol

In recent years, technological innovation and increased commercial interest have made alcohol testing in the workplace simpler. Among organisations that test employees for alcohol misuse at work, the most common approach is to test when an employee is suspected of alcohol misuse as a result of work performance or inappropriate behaviour, namely

---

> **Box 4.4 Key elements of a workplace alcohol policy**
>
> The key elements outlined below are based on common themes drawn from several current policies. Those offering policy templates routinely advise consultation with relevant stakeholders and legal advice in the context of organisational needs:
>
> - Clear rules on the use of alcohol in the work setting and its potential impact on work performance
> - An assessment of work-based influences on alcohol use and a commitment to remedying
> - Pointers to the potential dangers to the health and safety of drinkers and their colleagues
> - Investigation of instances where alcohol use may be implicated in poor performance, and appropriate action taken
> - Alcohol misuse considered as a health issue, with wide-ranging impact
> - Alcohol policies should be designed to assure problem drinkers that they will be treated fairly and encourage them to seek assistance, where appropriate
> - Provision of assistance and referral to appropriate services
> - The policy should apply to all workers
> - Suspension of disciplinary action in cases of misconduct or poor performance, where an alcohol problem is a factor, on condition that the worker follows a suitable course of action
> - Where gross misconduct is involved, an alcohol problem may be taken into account when determining disciplinary action
> - Paid leave or time off for problem drinking treatment

'for cause' testing. Random testing in the workplace is rare in the UK, occurring in about 10% of those companies who test. The Trades Union Congress (TUC) considers testing only appropriate for staff in safety-critical settings, and it believes testing should be part of a comprehensive safety strategy, including support and treatment for those who test positive (TUC: http://www.tuc.org.uk/ workplace/drugsandalcohol.cfm (accessed 12 August 2013)). A Chartered Institute of Personnel and Development (CIPD) (2007) survey showed that 22% of responding organisations tested employees for drugs or alcohol misuse, a modest increase on earlier 2001 findings. Of those questioned, 9% of organisations planned to introduce testing. Fifty-three percent of safety-critical organisations test, with a further 18% planning to do so. Of note, 65% of employers did not test and had no plans to do so. As these survey results are based on a 5% response rate, the views of non-responding employing organisations (95%) are unknown, and it may be concluded that, in the UK, testing in the workplace is a relatively uncommon practice. Drug testing can have an important role in safety-critical and other occupations where the public is entitled to expect the highest standards of safety and integrity; however, there is no justification for drug testing as a means of policing the private behaviour of employees, nor is it an appropriate tool for dealing with most performance issues (Independent Inquiry into Drug Testing at Work (UK) IIDTW, 2004; TUC: http://www.tuc.org.uk/workplace/drugsandalcohol.cfm (accessed 13 April 2013)). The reluctance of UK employers to test reflects prevailing cultural norms on alcohol and privacy as well as economic expediency. Generally, good management is considered the most effective method of improving workplace performance and tackling alcohol problems amongst staff and is preferred over testing (IIDTW, 2004).

Alcohol brief interventions and raising awareness in the workplace

Employment settings are common public health targets because the workforce represents a captive audience, there are similarities in employee characteristics, and the set of alcohol-related consequences (accidents, absenteeism) are specific to that organisation. Therefore, information and awareness campaigns, including brief interventions for hazardous and harmful drinkers, are commonly delivered by trained HR personnel and/or NHS health improvement professionals.

There is a significant body of evidence supporting the use of alcohol brief interventions (ABIs), which is discussed more fully in Chapter 6. However, the application and evaluation of ABIs in the workplace in the UK is rare. In a trial of public sector employees receiving ABI, these employees reported reduced alcohol consumption and fewer days' use of hospital services compared with those in a control group. This suggests that brief interventions in the workplace have the potential to reduce alcohol harm and also save resources. Additionally, more than 90% of respondents indicated that they had been happy to participate in a health and lifestyle survey. Some commented that the survey had raised their awareness of the risks associated with alcohol use and that they had found the information useful (Watson et al., 2009).

Opposing perspectives

Employers and their representative organisations appear less concerned about workplace alcohol issues.

An absence and workplace health survey (CBI, 2011) was conducted with human resource practitioners and managers in 223 organisations, in both public and private sectors. Respondent organisations employed just over 1 million people, representing approximately 4% of employees in the UK. The researchers concluded that health issues were viewed as the most common reason for poor performance at work, and non-work-related mental health issues were noted as the most common reason for long-term absence. However, alcohol is not mentioned in the survey findings though it is highly likely that alcohol is a factor in both poor work performance and non-work-related mental health issues.

The study by the Chartered Institute for Personnel and Development (2007) further illustrates the apparent indifference of employers to alcohol issues in the workplace, whether in relation to employee wellbeing, efficiency or productivity. The CIPD *Managing Drug and Alcohol Misuse at Work* survey (2007) is based on responses from over 500 UK-based human resource professionals working in organisations with a total of more than 1.1 million employees. However, the findings and the conclusions drawn are severely diluted as those respondents represent only 5% of the total number (around 10,000) of survey questionnaires distributed to HR practitioners. The low response may suggest that the topic of alcohol in the workplace is not high priority even though the findings from the 5% who responded have been used to illustrate a significant problem.

Alcohol Concern reported a study of FTSE 250 (Financial Times and Stock Exchange or 'footsie') companies, reviewing published reports and contacting human resource departments, and concluded that these companies are refusing to confront or acknowledge the problem. A little more than 20% of these companies had alcohol policies that featured obvious restrictions on being drunk at work, suggesting that most companies (78%) were ignoring alcohol as a workplace issue. A small minority (3.2%) had no plans to introduce such policies, including some who would only do so if legally required. These findings imply that there is a need for proper awareness and behaviour programmes to tackle the issues, and these programmes are increasingly important if British companies are to survive and thrive during difficult economic times. As a result of these findings, the UK government should include alcohol policy as a specific requirement under the Corporate Governance Code (Alcohol Concern, 2013).

The poor provision of alcohol policies in the workplace means that only 14% of UK workers have access to comprehensive occupational health services. Only 3% of companies offer a high level of provision; thus, the UK does not meet the minimum legal requirements of the European-wide Health and Safety Framework Directive (Hillier et al., 2005). If employers are unenthusiastic, this casts doubt on the feasibility of the EU (EAHF, 2011) proposals for collaborative partnerships to deal with workplace issues associated with alcohol.

! Thinking Point

Why do you think some employers appear reluctant to deal with alcohol issues in the workplace?

Summary Points

(1) The family has a major influence on young people's drinking, and a wide range of family issues contribute to hazardous drinking in young people, including excessive parental alcohol consumption. Alcohol problems run in families.

(2) The family is affected by the harmful drinking of one or more family members. Family discord and domestic violence are strongly associated with excessive drinking.

(3) A parent's or caregiver's alcohol consumption is a significant factor in child welfare and protection.

(4) Family plays an important role in recovery from alcohol problems.

(5) Some services focus specifically on the needs of wider family members to the exclusion of the drinker.

(6) Family-focused interventions have been demonstrated to reduce stress among family members and, in some instances, increase the likelihood of the drinker seeking help.

(7) Whole family approaches to problem drinking are effective in supporting change.

(8) The prevailing pro-alcohol culture is lenient towards alcohol and workplace issues.

(9) Loss of employment or the threat of redundancy is associated with heavy alcohol consumption.

(10) The workplace may be negatively affected by hazardous or harmful drinking, including safety, efficiency, attendance, sickness absence.

(11) Forces external to the workplace that influence alcohol consumption and drinking patterns (see Chapter 3) have an impact on the workforce. Workplace characteristics may also influence the impact of alcohol.

(12) The existence of restrictions on alcohol in the workplace and policies designed to deal with the problems of performance and absence receive wide support from public health bodies.

(13) Despite significant evidence of the impact of alcohol on the workplace, many employers appear reluctant to consider or implement workplace policies. This will limit the impact of the EU strategy, which requires an interdisciplinary approach that includes employers and other stakeholders.

(14) Alcohol policies should be included with other employee wellbeing strategies in the workplace. The presence and implementation of a workplace policy on alcohol sends a message to employees about acceptable conduct and reduces alcohol use, both at work and outside the work setting.

(15) Effective supervision and management of staff performance is important in both the prevention and identification of alcohol issues in the workplace and, in many instances, is a more effective response than substance use testing.

(16) Testing may be part of a workplace policy on a 'for cause' basis though, for some, it should only be used in safety-critical work settings.

(17) Targeting the workforce by raising alcohol awareness and conducting ABIs has been shown to have significant potential.

Web pages and resources

http://www.alcoholandfamilies.org.uk/documents/7/lit_
review/alcohol_family_problems.htm
*This page provides a review of the literature on alcohol
abuse and its impact on families.*

www.alcoholconcern.org.uk/publications/factsheets/
grasping-the-nettle
*Galvani (2010). Grasping the nettle: alcohol and
domestic violence. Factsheet. An excellent and brief
outline of alcohol and domestic violence as it impacts on
partners and children of problem drinkers: includes policy
and practice guidance.*

*UK national and regional bodies: These agencies outline
the arguments for action on alcohol in the work setting
and commonly provide guidance, training, and
education and sample workplace policies.*

http://www.alcoholconcern.org.uk/workplace
Alcohol Concern Web page on alcohol and the workplace.

www.hse.gov.uk/pubns/indg240.pdf
*Health and Safety Executive (HSE). Don't mix it. A
guide for employers on alcohol at work.*

http://www.scotland.gov.uk/Resource/0041/00416890.
doc
The Scottish government's model alcohol policy.

http://www.tuc.org.uk/workplace/drugsandalcohol.cfm
*The Trades Union Congress' (TUC) advice on alcohol in
the workplace.*

Further reading

Tobutt, C. (Ed.), 2011. Alcohol at Work: Managing
Alcohol Problems and Issues in the Workplace.
Gower, London.
*Current key text on this subject with the main themes
developed in detail.*

Valentine, G., et al., 2010. Alcohol consumption and
family life. Joseph Rowntree. www.jrf.org.uk.
*This is a report of a study that examined how parents
teach young children (5–12 years old) about alcohol. It
explored parental attitudes towards alcohol and family
drinking practices.*

Copello, A., Orford, J., 2002. Addiction and the family: is
it time for services to take notice of the evidence?
Addiction 97, 1361–1363.
*This paper outlines the evidence for the effectiveness of
family-focused interventions, many of which are outlined
in this chapter. Service providers are challenged to adopt a
family perspective, taking account of both need and
effectiveness.*

Copello, A., Orford, J., Hodgson, R., Tober, G., 2009.
Social Behaviour and Network Therapy for Alcohol
Problems. Routledge, East Sussex.
*This is the first manual on SBNT for those working with
people with alcohol problems. SBNT was evaluated in the
UK Alcohol Treatment Trial. This manual is easy to use
and practice-oriented.*

5   Public health interventions

There has been a significant shift in the UK government's stance on alcohol over the past three decades. The current view is that cheap alcohol is too readily available and industry needs and commercial advantages have been given priority over community concerns (DoH, 2012a,b). This chapter considers the three main alcohol control measures: minimum unit pricing, control of the drinking environment via liquor licensing and education. Each measure's primary function is prevention, with the aim of preventing or delaying the uptake of drinking. Similarly, all three measures may also have a secondary function: to reduce the harm to current users. In particular, the price of alcohol and its physical availability interact, given that individuals drink when and if they can afford it and not simply because sale outlets are open.

The price of alcohol

Alcohol pricing and taxation is a contentious topic, where the vested interests of the alcohol production and sale industries, individual liberty and state intervention collide. Governments frequently use the regulation of price and taxation on alcohol to raise revenue to support a variety of expenditures, and, in some countries, this regulation has been used to minimise harm. In general, studies show that increases in price and tax on alcohol reduce consumption and the associated alcohol-related health and social consequences, whereas cheaper alcohol results in increased consumption and greater harm.

Affordability

In the UK, alcohol was 66% more affordable in 2009 compared to 1987 (ISD, 2011). This has come about because, while the price of alcohol increased more than the general retail prices of other commodities, household disposable income increased substantially more during that period. Also, during the same period, alcohol purchased from off-sales (off-licences, shops, and supermarkets) has become considerably more affordable than on-trade (pubs, clubs and hotels). In 2009, beer was 155% more affordable when bought from off-sales compared to 39% more affordable from licensed premises. During the same period, spirits and wine combined became 50% more affordable from licensed premises and 126% more affordable from off-licensed premises (ISD, 2011).

Price mechanisms and consumption

Alcoholic beverages, like any other commodity, are influenced by the rules of supply and demand. A limited supply and constant or increased demand will result in high alcohol prices. The same high level of demand with unlimited supply or decreased demand with a constant supply will result in low alcohol prices. The potential for price and taxation to

be manipulated will, in turn, affect the relationships between supply and demand. Central to the use of price as a means of controlling purchase, and by implication consumption, is the concept of price elasticity of demand. This predicts the extent to which a given price change will result in a change in consumption and is defined as the percentage change in consumption resulting from a 1% change in price. Inelastic demand refers to stable demand or consumption in the face of increased price; it is useful for revenue generation schemes, as consumption remains unchanged while price and, in turn, revenues may be increased.

Table 5.1 shows the results of a systematic review demonstrating the mean price elasticity of alcoholic beverages and consequent reductions in per capita consumption on the basis of a 10% increase in beverage price. Mean elasticity scores vary from one

Table 5.1 Mean elasticity scores and reductions in consumption following 10% price increase

BEVERAGE	MEAN ELASTICITY SCORE	PRICE INCREASE (%)	REDUCTION IN CONSUMPTION (%)	NUMBER OF SUPPORTING STUDIES
Beer	−0.46	10	4.6	105
Wine	−0.69	10	6.9	93
Spirits	−0.80	10	8.0	103
Alcohol (overall)	−0.51	10	5.1	91
Heavy alcohol use	−0.28	10	2.8	10

Source: Wagenaar et al. (2009).

beverage to another. This score is aggregated for all alcoholic beverages. Alcoholic beverages are relatively inelastic in that a 10% increase in price results in a decrease in consumption, irrespective of beverage type. Price elasticity is lower for alcoholic beverages among heavy alcohol users, whose consumption is affected by price changes to a lesser extent than that of the population as a whole. Larger reductions in consumption would require further price increases.

Because the mean elasticity scores are based on a large number of studies, the price elasticity of specific beverages does not necessarily equate to any single country. Therefore, price elasticity for beverages in the UK, for example, might vary from those in Table 5.1. Furthermore, within the UK, there may be regional variations in elasticity for particular beverages, which reflect a range of cultural factors. Consequently, estimates of tax and price effects also reflect particular meanings and uses of alcoholic beverages across diverse social and cultural environments, and tax and price policies probably interact with a whole web of individual, community and social influences on drinking behaviour (Wagenaar et al., 2009, p. 189).

Many governments, on the basis of a variety of influences, including vested interests, are reluctant to raise taxes on alcohol. The stability of these taxes over time results in inflation eroding their value and a decline in the real price of alcohol. However, Wagenaar et al.

(2009) conclude that the relatively inelastic demand for alcohol will result in reductions in consumption as well as the potential to sustain or increase revenue. Babor et al. (2003) argue that the responsiveness of alcohol consumption to its price affects not only the efficiency with which special alcohol taxes generate revenue but also the potential health benefits to be reaped from higher alcohol prices. In this sense, the purposes of a public health approach and a revenue-raising strategy are both served. In a systematic review of 112 studies, researchers noted highly significant relationships between alcohol tax or price measures, alcohol sales and self-reported consumption. They concluded that there is overwhelming evidence of the effects that alcohol prices have on drinking. Wagenaar et al. (2009) found that price affects drinking of all types of beverages, and, across the population of drinkers from light drinkers to heavy drinkers and at the most basic level, price interacts with income to affect consumption. These findings provide a strong rationale for using increases in alcoholic beverage taxes to promote public health by reducing drinking.

However, the relative price of alcohol may be influenced by factors other than public health or revenue-raising strategies. Consequently, alcohol consumption has reduced since 2005 in response to economic changes, such as rising costs of living, restrictions on wage increases and job losses.

Price change and altered consumption and harm

There have been a number of studies that report the impact of price change. In Alaska in both 1983 and 2002, alcoholic beverage tax increases reduced alcohol-related disease mortality significantly, including deaths from liver cirrhosis, acute alcohol poisoning, alcohol-related cancers, and cardiovascular diseases (Chaloupka, 2009). Reductions in physical abuse of spouses, children and other violent behaviours as a result of increases in alcohol pricing and taxation were also noted (Chaloupka, 2009). Giesbrecht et al. (2010) note the impact of consumption levels and the effects of drinking on families and communities.

Taxes on alcohol were reduced in Finland in 2004, a country where the high price of alcohol was a cornerstone of an effective public health strategy. An association between the tax cuts and an increase of 17% in the number of sudden deaths involving alcohol in the previous year was noted (Koski et al., 2007). This reflected increases in alcohol consumption and alcohol-related consequences (Holder, 2007). In a review of alcohol taxation, Makela and Osterberg (2009) concluded that the reductions in alcohol taxes in Finland in 2004 had the most significant effect on the poorer section of the population in terms of health damage due to reductions in alcohol prices and consequent increased consumption.

In 1980, the duty on alcohol was increased in the UK, resulting in an increase in the real cost of alcohol for the first time in several decades. From 1979 to 1981, Kendell et al. (1983) conducted interviews with over 400 regular drinkers in Scotland, before and after the price increase, giving researchers an opportunity to assess the impact of the price change on levels of consumption and alcohol problems. The price increase resulted in marked decreases in alcohol consumption as well as reported levels of alcohol-related problems. Importantly, it also demonstrated that heavy drinkers also reduced their consumption. In a survey of harmful drinkers in Edinburgh, it was found that average consumption was almost 200 units of alcohol in the previous week. They reported buying alcohol at, on average, 43 pence and as low as 9 pence per unit. The lower the price, the more they consumed, and cheapness was commonly offered as the reason for choice of beverage. As harmful drinkers are generally heavy consumers of the cheapest alcohol available, it is suggested that increased price could have a relatively large impact on their consumption and, in turn, health (Black et al., 2011).

While the evidence of a connection between price and availability, consumption and harm is clear, those people with commercial interests in the production and sale of alcohol maintain an opposing view. They argue that restrictive measures on pricing, availability, advertising and marketing of alcohol are blunt, ineffective measures that affect only the moderate majority. They suggest that, instead of increasing taxes on alcohol, the government should educate consumers about drinking responsibly (Harkins and Poley, 2011).

Pricing policy options

Alcohol producers and marketers also suggest that increased taxation may not necessarily result in a price increase for the consumer because retailers, including supermarkets, may absorb the cost.

Taxation applied to alcoholic beverages bears little relation to alcohol content or potential harm, having evolved piecemeal for a variety of historical reasons (Donaldson and Rutter, 2011). Internationally, the policy approaches are diverse, and these policies have been proposed, implemented or modelled in relation to alcohol price regulation. These include:

Inflation linked taxation: The price of alcohol is linked to the rate of inflation. The cost of alcohol remains stable relative to other commodities and as a result consumption is regulated. Failure to link beverage alcohol price to inflation tends to result in cheaper alcohol and increased consumption.

Volumetric taxation: Tax on alcohol is based on alcohol content of the beverage. Thus, more tax would be paid on a bottle of spirits (40% alcohol by volume) compared to a bottle of wine (10–14% alcohol by volume).

Differential (targeted) taxation: Specific beverages are targeted, and taxes are

increased on only those beverages, for example, "alcopops" ciders. A German study concluded that drinkers switched from the targeted beverages to consuming spirits and expressed an increased preference for beverages associated with riskier drinking patterns (Muller et al., 2010).

Ban on price promotions: This option refers to restrictions on alcohol sales as loss leaders and promotional offers. This is broadly supported by the UK government and was implemented by the Scottish government in 2011.

Minimum unit pricing: The fixing of a minimum price for a unit of alcohol applied to the purchase of alcohol either on licensed premises (such as a public house or club) or off-licence premises (such as a supermarket or off-licence) (Booth et al., 2008; Meier et al., 2010). In the UK, the chief medical officers for all four countries support minimum pricing for alcohol; legislation related to minimum pricing has been passed by the Scottish government, and the UK government has indicated its intention to implement such pricing (DoH, 2012a,b).

The Sheffield Studies: Minimum unit price

In a review of pricing policies, Booth et al. (2008) concluded that there was limited understanding of the effects of pricing on different purchasing and consumption patterns among subgroups of the population. Studies of alcohol pricing policy options were commissioned by the

UK government to investigate the impact of alternative policies on priority groups, namely underage drinkers (under the age of 18), 18–24-year-old binge drinkers, and harmful drinkers (those consuming in excess of the recommended safe limits). The resulting research publications are widely known as the Sheffield Studies (Booth et al., 2008; Brennan et al., 2008; Meier et al., 2010).

In an economic modelling study designed to evaluate how price control options reduced harm at a general population level, Meier et al. (2010) measured the impact of differing policy options on different population subgroups. These studies were innovative in that they considered the heterogeneity of the population as an important dimension of effect and created the opportunity for policies to be more sophisticated and targeted (Room and Livingston, 2010). Subgroups were examined by age, gender and three consumption levels as well as beverage type, price and place of purchase. These studies showed that while alcohol policies may appear similar at a general population level, subgroups are affected differently by alternative policies.

Table 5.2 shows the alcohol pricing policy options that have the greatest impact. Policy options resulting in a 4%, or greater, reduction in consumption indicate the impact on particular target groups. A general price increase of 10% would reduce consumption in the total population between 4.4% and 6.0%, including all target groups, and these findings are consistent with Wagenaar et al.'s (2009) systematic review. The total population is clearly influenced by 40 and 50 pence minimum unit pricing as well as the general 10% price increase. The impact on the total population is less than the impact on the target groups, with the exception of hazardous drinkers less than 25 years old. The total population is not a proxy for the ordinary or moderate drinker because it includes those drinking at hazardous and harmful levels. Therefore, the impact of price changes on moderate drinkers would be less than the impact on the total population.

It is estimated that in the UK harmful drinkers, including those dependent on alcohol, would be most affected by minimum unit pricing at 40 or 50 pence per unit and a general 10% price increase. A total ban on off-trade discounting would have the greatest impact on women, whose consumption would reduce by 4.1%, reflecting the fact that women commonly buy alcohol from off-sales, including supermarkets. Hazardous drinkers under the age of 25 would be most affected by a minimum price of 30p (off-trade) and 80p (on-trade) or a price increase of 25% on low-price on-trade products, while the impact of minimum unit pricing at 40p per unit is ineffective and at 50p moderately effective in changing consumption. This reflects the extent to which younger people drink in pubs and other licensed premises.

Specific pricing policies would affect different groups in a variety of ways; this

Table 5.2 Percentage reduction in alcohol consumption for selected policy options: by drinker subgroup and gender

POLICY INTERVENTION	TOTAL POPULATION	HAZARDOUS DRINKERS	HAZARDOUS UNDER 25	HARMFUL DRINKERS	MALE	FEMALE
General price increase: 10%	4.4	4.7	6.0	4.5	4.4	4.4
Minimum price 50p	6.9	5.9	3.0	10.3	5.6	9.3
Minimum price 40p	2.6	1.8	0.7	4.5	2.2	3.5
Total ban off-trade discounting	2.8	3.1	0.9	3.2	2.1	4.1
Minimum price 30p/80p off-/on-trade	2.1	1.9	7.2	2.5	2.5	1.4
Low-price on-trade: 25% increase	0.6	0.2	6.1	1.1	0.4	0.9

Source: Meier et al. (2010).

fact indicates both the flexibility and sensitivity of such approaches on a range of population subgroups and their distinctive alcohol purchasing and consumption patterns.

Controlling drinking environments

A drinking occasion may involve drinking at home, in licensed premises, or other settings. Because the largest proportion of alcohol is purchased from off-sales, the community, including licensed premises and the family home, may also be considered to be drinking environments.

Liquor licensing

The Licensing (Scotland) Act of 1976, designed to reduce binge drinking and make licensed premises more family friendly, was a landmark piece of legislation for Scotland and the UK. The extended hours effectively introduced all-day and late-evening alcohol sales. Research into consumption patterns following the licensing changes was neutral in its findings (Duffy, 1992). This research, then, formed part of the argument to deregulate alcohol licensing in England and Wales in the mid to late 1980s, with deregulation and individual responsibility comprising the zeitgeist of the 1980s.

A review of Scottish liquor licensing described its remit as a balancing exercise, which took account of many serious causes for concern but also recognised other considerations, including public

preference and commercial interests (Nicholson, 2003). The licensing principles proposed by the Nicholson Report (2003) became cornerstones of the subsequent legislation: prevention of crime or disorder and public nuisance; promotion of public safety and public health; and protection of children from harm. Scottish licensing legislation was unique in prioritising public health. However, a public health dimension is now apparent in liquor licensing debates across the UK (DoH, 2012a,b).

The past decade has seen high-street off-licence chains in the UK, such as Threshers, all but disappear. Supermarkets now dominate wine sales, their economies of scale driving down prices and destroying much of the opposition (Williams, 2011).

Safer licensed premises

A tripartite relationship, involving self-regulation (of the licensed premises), formal enforcement (by police and licensing authorities), and the engagement of local community groups (in consultation and decision making) has been proposed as a means of reducing harm (Homel et al., 2004).

Licensed premises (pubs, clubs) are a focus of alcohol-related offences, including violence, despite the overall decrease in the purchase of alcohol in these settings. Pubs and clubs where alcohol-related aggression and violence occur are often crowded, have frustrated customers because of slow service, poor ventilation, and a lax approach to age limits. Creating a safer licensed drinking environment is essentially a regulatory matter where formal enforcement of regulations is required but is not in itself sufficient (Stockwell and Gruenewald, 2004). Effective regulation should ensure that the physical environment is attractive; sends a message to patrons about appropriate behaviour; and does not irritate people by being crowded, excessively noisy, hot, or smoky (Homel et al., 2004, p. 235). Furthermore, serving staff should be trained appropriately and should not tolerate drunkenness. Paradoxically, some of the features of risky licensed premises are precisely what make them attractive to some drinkers. Thus, harmful and dependent drinkers may benefit from licensed premises where behaviour is controlled by staff and fellow drinkers (Black et al., 2011).

Age restriction

Age restrictions on the sale of alcohol are intended to protect young people by limiting access to alcohol in order to prevent alcohol problems. While it is against the law in the UK for someone 18 or over to purchase alcohol for someone under the age of 18, it is not illegal for someone under the age of 18 to consume alcohol. It is, however, against the law in the UK to give alcohol to a child under 5 years of age.

There is a consistent body of research on the impact of public drinking-age laws and alcohol-related consequences. Amendments to the legal drinking age result in changes in a range of problems associated with intoxication, such as road traffic fatalities, serious assault, crime, and drunkenness. A higher legal drinking age has been shown to result in fewer alcohol-related consequences (Wagenaar, 1993).

A legal reduction of the drinking age from 21 to 18 in Western Australia resulted in a substantial increase in rates for serious assaults when compared with Queensland where the age restriction remained in place (Stockwell and Gruenewald, 2004).

Proposals by the Scottish government to restrict off-sales to those age 21 and over met with opposition. The Scottish Youth Parliament argued that the proposals were misguided and discriminatory (Braiden, 2011). Public opinion on age restrictions is usually divided, and age limits are difficult to change (Stockwell and Gruenewald, 2004). Rigorous enforcement of licensing laws and age restrictions has a beneficial effect on underage drinking and associated negative consequences. There is broad support for the enforcement of current underage drinking laws, which may achieve as much as an unpopular increase in the legal drinking age.

Permitted opening hours

Afternoon closure of licensed premises disappeared during the 1980s, following liberalisation of liquor licensing across the UK. In general, increased trading hours are associated with a higher incidence of alcohol-related harm and vice versa (Raistrick et al., 1999).

The main interest in permitted hours concerns control of the negative consequences of night-time drinking. In New South Wales, Australia, pub closing times were restricted to 3 am, resulting in a 37% reduction in assaults in the city of Newcastle, compared to Hamilton where the restriction was not imposed (Kypri et al., 2010). Overall, opening hours tend to influence the timing of drunkenness and associated problems. Very late opening is associated with relatively higher levels of violence and road traffic accidents. Alcohol-related consequences may be reduced by shorter hours and even closure of outlets on certain days (Babor et al., 2003). Such findings contradict the ethos of licensing and attitudes towards alcohol in the UK. In Scotland, Nicholson (2003) recommended that permitted opening hours should be abolished and that there should be no statutorily prohibited hours. Fourteen hours per day was considered reasonable, with the onus being on the licensee to demonstrate appropriate opening hours to the licensing board. A similar approach was adopted for England and Wales, in the Licensing Act 2003, which permitted 24-hour openings. There is no evidence that these changes resulted in reductions in alcohol-related harm. The Police Reform and Social Responsibility Act (2011) covered a rebalancing of prior legislation (though permitted hours remained unchanged), which consisted of:

- doubling the fine for persistent underage sales to £20,000
- introducing a late-night levy to help cover the cost of policing the late-night alcohol sales economy
- increasing the flexibility of early morning alcohol-restriction orders
- lowering the evidential threshold on licensing authorities
- removing the vicinity test for licensing representations to allow wider local community involvement
- reforming the system of temporary event notices (TENs)
- suspension of premises licences due to non-payment of annual fees (Home Office, 2011)

Policies to restrict drunkenness and antisocial behaviour

Since the 1970s, there have been a variety of policies and practices designed to reduce alcohol-related antisocial behaviour. In response to public concerns about antisocial behaviour, there appears to be a shift toward criminalising the drinker (Rodger, 2008).

Off-sales

An off-sales licence is granted for the sale of alcohol which is consumed off the premises, for example, at licensed grocers, supermarkets, and off-sales establishments. Like pubs, some off-licences are the focus of antisocial behaviour. In a review of off-sales in the community (Scottish Government, 2003), the off-sales referred to were corner shop establishments where the connections between purchase, consumption and disorderly conduct were clear; there was no discussion of large supermarkets as off-sales. Dedicated off-sales and licensed grocers were most frequently used by young people to obtain alcohol. Family grocers were less likely to have training to prevent illegal sales and may be more vulnerable to pressure and threats. Better engagement and consultation about granting licences was sought at the community level, and communities felt that police should give greater priority to responding to antisocial behaviour (DoH, 2012a,b).

Public drinking bans

Restrictions on drinking in public places are designed to reduce the potential for drunkenness and antisocial behaviour. Many towns and cities across the UK have adopted bans on drinking in public, so that any person who consumes alcohol in a designated place or is found to be in possession of an open container in a designated place shall be guilty of an offence (www.glasgow.gov.uk). The offence is essentially possession and/or consumption, not necessarily drunkenness. A rise in offences might be explained by the increase of such laws rather than a real increase in offending.

Fixed penalty notices

The introduction of fixed penalty notices (FPNs) in Scotland was designed to enable police to deal with antisocial

behaviours in the night-time economy, while maintaining police presence on the street. A large proportion of FPNs issued are for alcohol-related nuisances. Around 80% of police officers surveyed considered that most of the individuals given FPNs were under the influence of alcohol, and the officers were divided on whether FPNs would reduce antisocial behaviour (Scottish Government, 2009).

Drinking banning orders

Drinking banning orders (DBOs) are intended to tackle alcohol-related criminal or disorderly behaviour and to protect others affected. The order can last from 2 months to 2 years and is available to the court through the Violent Crime Reduction Act (2006) in England and Wales. An order can be made against a person age 16 or over if they engage in criminal or disorderly behaviour while under the influence of alcohol and the court considers it necessary to protect the public. Police (including British Transport Police) and local authorities can apply to the courts for an order. The legislation enables courts to offer education on the health and social consequences of heavy alcohol consumption to those subject to a DBO, on a voluntary basis. A DBO may impose any prohibition on a person that the court considers necessary to protect others. This could include exclusion from buying alcohol, consuming alcohol or being in possession of alcohol in public. Further restrictions may also include individual or sets of licensed premises or all licensed premises in a geographical area.

Drunk and incapable

In addition to dealing with alcohol-fuelled antisocial behaviour, police and the health service in the UK deal with those who are drunk and incapable. This includes those drunk on a single occasion, so-called binge drinkers who present on several occasions and chronic recidivists who are possibly alcohol dependent. The practices involved in the delivery of sobriety services vary greatly, reflecting local needs, and involving triage, first aid, custody nurses, cell monitoring, ambulance and police protocols, accident and emergency services and mobile services in city centres (Griesbach et al., 2009). Box 5.1 lists the proposed local actions in the policy agenda outlined in the UK government's Alcohol Strategy (DoH, 2012a,b).

Outlet density

In British Columbia, Canada, alcohol sales were investigated in relation to increased outlet density. A policy of privatisation resulted in a 100% increase in private alcohol outlets, and the greater number of private outlets, as opposed to government liquor stores, was associated with higher per capita consumption (Stockwell et al., 2009).

Box 5.1 Proposed local action: England and Wales

- Powers to reduce harm: changes to public health; new Police and Crime Commissioners.
- Rebalancing the Licensing Act; health-related objective for alcohol licensing.
- Restrict alcohol sales late at night through extended powers to introduce Early Morning Restriction Orders.
- Power to introduce a new late-night levy: businesses that sell alcohol into the late night contribute to the cost of policing.
- Pilot sobriety schemes: removing the right to drink from those who have shown they cannot drink responsibly.
- Control the outlet density.
- £1m to help local agencies and businesses tackle problem drinking.
- Conduct a pilot study to provide further information on crime occurring on or near local alcohol hotspots.
- Develop new injunctions as part of the response to antisocial behaviour. Explore giving NHS Protect the power to apply for these injunctions.
- Encourage hospitals to share non-confidential information about alcohol-related injuries with police and other local agencies.

Source: DoH (2012a,b, p. 16).

In Melbourne, Australia, an association between outlet density and domestic violence and assault was recorded for pubs (and other on-premise licences), and there was a stronger association for off-sales. Livingston (2011) suggests that licensing policies need to pay more attention to off-licence outlets, including supermarkets. The relationship between outlet density and domestic violence and other alcohol-related consequences reflects aspects of the community and its social make-up (Leonard, 2011). Organised neighbourhoods, whether reflecting social class or level of community activism, may be more effective at reducing or preventing an increase in alcohol outlets. Disadvantaged communities are commonly less able to influence policies to their benefit. A stable neighbourhood or community may withstand an increase in outlets without a subsequent increase in negative consequences. Additionally, transitory neighbourhoods may be more affected by increased outlet density, particularly off-sales outlets, and, in turn, have increased prevalence of harm. A younger, less-conforming neighbourhood population might attract greater police attention, leading to increased reports of family violence, independent of the impact of outlet density on consumption or harm.

While outlet density is indirectly related to health and social problems, policy guidance (Scottish Government, 2007; DoH, 2012a,b) only notes the importance of outlet density but does not provide an ideal number of outlets in a community. The duty of determining the number of outlets per community has fallen to the local licensing authority. The increased democratisation of the licensing process is important, in that community organisations can be involved at the planning and complaint stages. However, a lack of community activity or concern may result in licensing decisions that adversely affect a community.

Alcohol education

An educational approach toward preventing alcohol misuse is supported and promoted by the UK government and the alcohol industry (DoE, 2012) for a number of reasons. First, if alcohol problems reflect inequality in society, then alcohol education is much cheaper to create and disseminate than rebalancing the social inequalities, and politicians can demonstrate that something has been done about the problem. Second, the alcohol production and sales industry often contributes to educational programmes (perhaps in order to demonstrate their civic mindedness), which allows commercial interests to flourish and may increase their public profiles. Finally, the general public consider education to be an approach that fits with broader societal values. In cultures based on educational development and attainment, the continued delivery of alcohol education represents a marker of public concern.

> ### Box 5.2 Levels of alcohol education
>
> Primary prevention: Prevent drinking by supporting abstinence, but more commonly by delaying the uptake.
>
> Secondary prevention: Reduce heavy drinking and drunkenness (binge drinking) among those already drinking.
>
> Harm reduction: Reduce harms associated with drinking, without necessarily focusing on consumption. This approach runs the risk of appearing to condone drinking.
>
> Settings: classroom, family, whole school, and community.

Box 5.2 gives an overview of the levels of alcohol education.

Evidence of effectiveness of alcohol education

While it is reasonable to think that education should be one of the most effective interventions, there is limited evidence of its effectiveness. There is no consensus as to which prevention approach offers the greatest benefit and even whether there is any benefit at all. Neither giving information nor enhancing personal development are effective in preventing or delaying alcohol use. Social learning theory purports that young people are susceptible to social influences to use alcohol. Therefore, awareness of these influences, including normative information on drinking by young people, the development of general social skills, and the development of specific skills to resist temptation to drink form the basis of education about social influences.

There is strong appeal in the engagement of family and school and community approaches that offer reinforcement of messages delivered in a time-limited classroom setting. The community may feel good about delivering strong anti-drug or anti-alcohol messages, but any programme that does not change behaviour is a waste of resources and fails in its responsibility to young people (Midford, 2010).

Systematic reviews of alcohol education as a preventive intervention

In a systematic review (Foxcroft et al., 2002), almost 40% of programmes reviewed showed evidence of ineffectiveness. Those that reported longer-term evaluations (over 3 years follow-up) were examined. The Strengthening Families Programme in particular, but also culturally focused skills training, showed promise. All studies reviewed showed some methodological weaknesses and replication with more robust designs was recommended.

In a systematic review of alcohol misuse prevention programmes for children and adolescents, Foxcroft and Tsertsvadze (2011) examined the effectiveness of school-based, family-based, and multi-component programmes by considering randomised controlled trials. They concluded that most family-based programmes were effective, while multi-component programmes showed insufficient evidence of additional benefit. However, they cautioned that bias and/or contextual factors may have affected trial results.

School-based programmes: In school settings, prevention programmes commonly took the form of alcohol awareness education, social and peer resistance skills, normative feedback (on peers' consumption), or the development of behavioural norms and positive peer-group affiliation. These approaches were delivered as school lessons or behaviour-management programmes or workshops.

Family-based programmes: In family settings, the prevention programmes commonly took the form of developing parental skills and offering support, nurturing behaviours, the establishment of rules and boundaries, and subsequent monitoring. Some elements of the school-based programmes were also incorporated in some studies, such as development of behavioural norms and peer affiliation. Most of the family-oriented studies reported in systematic reviews recorded small but positive effects, which persisted over the medium to long term (Smit et al., 2008; Foxcroft and Tsertsvadze, 2011).

The Örebro prevention programme (Sweden) is an interesting example of a family-based programme and also demonstrates some of the methodological difficulties involved in evaluation (Holder, 2010). This parent-focused intervention was found to halve the increase in the frequency of drunkenness in 13–16 year olds, including high-risk pupils who had been drunk at age 13. Medium to large reductions in criminal or antisocial behaviour were reported. As hypothesised, the programme seemed to work by maintaining strict anti-drinking norms among parents. It was concluded that working via parents was an effective way to reduce underage drinking as well as delinquency (Koutsakis et al., 2008). However, independent replication failed to support the original findings and concluded that the programme did not appear to reduce or delay youthful drunkenness, that the significant difference in drunkenness was due to drop-out by heavier drinkers and failure to account for families that were not followed up. Furthermore, the apparent impact on parental attitudes and behaviour may have been due to parents and children being more likely to give the responses approved by the programme. The Örebro programme joins other prevention programmes found effective when tested by their designers but which later failed to show an effect when evaluated independently. It is possible that the enthusiasm and expertise of the designers, who were also the evaluators, was communicated to the parents (Bodin and Strandberg, 2011). However, the original trial did demonstrate the potential for parental involvement and for the school to be a source of reinforcement for parental responsibility regarding young people's drinking in a culture that accepts such messages. This is consistent with other studies.

Multi-component education programmes: Multi-component programmes were defined as those delivered in multiple settings, such as both school and family. There is evidence that multi-component interventions for alcohol misuse prevention can be effective, but there is insufficient evidence to conclude that multi-component programmes have any additional benefit compared to a single-component programme.

Certain generic, as opposed to alcohol-specific, psychosocial and developmental prevention programmes appeared effective and could be considered in relation to policy and practice. The evidence supports the effectiveness of certain universal prevention programmes (school, family, multi-component) that tend not to focus on the prevention of one particular behaviour but are designed to influence a range of health and lifestyle activities such as smoking, alcohol, sex, diet and mental health. Therefore, these programmes have the potential to influence a broader set of problem behaviours, as opposed to alcohol-specific prevention initiatives.

Important methodological limitations and reporting problems were identified, though improvements were noted in comparison to previous systematic reviews (Foxcroft and Tsertsvadze, 2011). Studies on family-based prevention of alcohol misuse in young people were weak on generalisablility of findings and health and social implications (Fernandez-Hermida et al., 2012).

Guidance for alcohol education

The National Institute for Health and Clinical Excellence (NICE) produced public health guidance for primary and secondary schools and other educational establishments, including further education, on sensible alcohol consumption (NICE, 2007). This guidance is designed for those with a remit in health and wellbeing working in education and the health service, local authorities and the wider public, as well as voluntary and community sectors, and this guidance is consistent with guidance in the rest of the UK. NICE (2007) states that school-based alcohol interventions were found to be cost-effective as they may avert the high costs associated with harmful drinking. However, it also indicated that the economic analysis carried out was subject to very large uncertainties. Given the limited impact that alcohol education has in changing drinking behaviour, the cost effectiveness of such an approach must remain open to question. See Box 5.3 for

---

Box 5.3 NICE Guidance (2007) School-based education and advice: main recommendations

Recommendation 1

Target population: Children and young people in schools (universal).

Action

- ensure alcohol education is an integral part of the national curriculum, Department Education guidance (England and Wales).
- ensure alcohol education is tailored for age, stage and learning needs.
- aim to encourage children *not* to drink, *delay* the age at which young people start drinking, and *reduce harm* among those who drink.
- programmes should:
  - increase knowledge of potential damage
  - explore attitudes to alcohol
  - help develop decision making, assertiveness, coping and verbal/non-verbal skills
  - help develop self-esteem
  - increase awareness of how the media, advertisements, role models, parents, peers and society can influence alcohol consumption.
- introduce a "whole school" approach to alcohol.
- offer parents or carers information about parenting skills, setting boundaries and resisting peer pressure.

Recommendation 2

Target population: Children and young people in schools, thought to be drinking harmfully.

Action

- offer brief, one-to-one advice; reduce the risks; and inform students where to find sources of support: this is akin to ABI (see Chapter 6 for further details on brief interventions).
- offer follow-up consultations or refer to external services.
- follow best practice on child protection, consent and confidentiality; where appropriate, involve parents or carers.

recommendations from the NICE guidelines.

Those at risk (and whose parents, carers or family members misuse alcohol) should be targeted (DoE,

2012). These individuals may include those who endure social deprivation, have poor school attendance, have family problems, and may be known to Children and Family Services

Summary Points

1. An increase in the price of alcohol will generally result in reduced consumption and related harm. Conversely, a reduction in the cost will result in increased consumption and harm.

2. Public health measures to reduce consumption and governments' desire to raise income are not mutually exclusive and may make price control more palatable to governments.

3. The economic model underpinning the Sheffield Studies demonstrates the potential to design alcohol price controls, which account for the heterogeneity of the population where the impact is greater than in the total population and among moderate drinkers, including minimum unit pricing.

4. The impact of current price regulation proposals is modest when compared to the large increases in per capita consumption and harm since the 1980s.

5. The pricing of alcohol as a means of reducing harm appears to be firmly on political agendas across the UK.

6. Licensing controls reflect a balance between community, health and commercial interests.

7. There is an emerging public health agenda underpinning liquor licensing. However, research findings on reductions in consequences (reduced opening hours, legal drinking age) are contrary to the ethos of licensing across the UK.

8. Measures dealing with antisocial behaviour reflect a shift toward blaming and criminalising the drinker.

9. A tripartite arrangement (regulation of licensed premises, enforcement by licensing authorities and police, and engagement of community groups) is the optimum approach to reduce harm.

10. Prevention regulations directed toward commercial sellers and backed up with enforcement are more effective than prevention programmes relying solely on education or persuasion directed toward individual drinkers.

11. There is consistent evidence that social influence prevention programmes have a small but positive effect on drinking, whether school based or family based, by delaying the uptake of drinking and reducing drunkenness or harm.

12. Educating consumers, of whatever age, to drink responsibly may have limited effectiveness when the prevailing culture and commercial interests act in opposition.

13. Alcohol education is broadly supported by government and the alcohol industry. As an approach, it is best combined in a package of public health approaches as opposed to a stand-alone preventive intervention.

Continued

14. Easy availability of low-price alcohol is likely to support pro-alcohol attitudes among peers, family and the community.

15. Regulatory arrangements are more effective than persuasion or education. Control of availability of alcohol by price is the most effective, and cheapest, method of reducing alcohol-related consequences. A variety of approaches to controlling the drinking environment, in its broadest sense, have been shown to be effective, though they are not necessarily consistent with current UK liquor licensing laws. There has been an increase in criminalising responses to alcohol-related disorder in public places.

and youth offending services. Education for young people whose drinking is identified as risky is akin to alcohol brief interventions (ABIs).

Web pages and resources

http://www.alcohol-focus-scotland.org.uk/minimum-pricing
Alcohol Focus Scotland web pages discussing minimum pricing of units of alcohol

http://www.nice.org.uk/nicemedia/pdf/PH007Guidance.pdf
The National Institute for Health and Clinical Excellence (2007) (NICE) publication, Intervention in schools to prevent and reduce alcohol use among children and young people

http://www.homeoffice.gov.uk/publications/alcohol-drugs/alcohol/alcohol-strategy?view=Binary
The UK Government Alcohol Strategy 2012

Further reading

Babor, T.F., et al., 2010. Alcohol: No Ordinary Commodity: Research and Public Policy. Oxford University Press, Oxford, UK.

6 Alcohol brief interventions (ABIs)

Alcohol brief interventions (ABIs) are a crucial addition to the strategies used to combat alcohol-related harm (Heather, 1994). ABIs are an element of public health and preventive responses that reflect the broadening of the concept of alcohol-related problems beyond the narrow focus on dependence or addiction; therefore, ABIs are based on the notion of targeting large populations of hazardous and harmful drinkers and intervening at an early stage. Given the significant numbers of drinkers who may participate in ABIs, substantial improvements in both individual and public health may be achieved.

Screening and brief interventions for alcohol-related problems represent an initial and opportunistic means of reviewing alcohol consumption and related harm among health care seekers. Brief interventions are consistent with a stepped care approach whereby individuals are offered the least intrusive intervention as a first step. Those with severe alcohol-related problems may be identified and offered referrals to appropriate services (Raistrick et al., 2006).

Identification of and screening for ABI

Screening questionnaires are usually available in printed or electronic formats, and they can be filled out by the client/patient, or the practitioner can read the questionnaire to the client/patient. Accuracy is enhanced when the questions are easily understood and clearly related to the service user's current health status. Practitioners should be non-judgemental in their approach, and the confidentiality of information provided should be assured. Additionally, if possible, the service user should be alcohol or drug free at the time. Screening questionnaires are presented in a self-report format and, as such, alcohol consumption and consequences may be over- or under-reported. However, it is widely agreed that these questionnaires are generally more accurate and economic to administer than assessing clinical indicators or biological measures (Raistrick et al., 2006).

The majority of health care patients participate in screening procedures on many health topics, such as diet and smoking, as part of routine practice. While ABIs may be offered on the basis of a lengthy health history or prior knowledge, the aim of an opportunistic intervention is to use brief screening questionnaires on large numbers of health service users routinely and rapidly to identify hazardous and harmful drinkers. All screening techniques listed in this chapter have tested positively for validity and reliability, indicating sensitivity (the proportion of hazardous or harmful drinkers who screened positive) and specificity (the proportion of non-hazardous or non-harmful drinkers who screened negative).

A significant number of screening questionnaires are used both in research and in practice settings. They are designed to identify hazardous, harmful or potentially dependent drinkers. Two distinct generations of alcohol screening questionnaires are commonly used: (1) those based on Cutting down, Annoyance by criticism, Guilty feeling and Eye-opener (CAGE) (Mayfield et al., 1974) and (2) those based on AUDIT (Alcohol Use Disorders Identification Test) (Babor et al., 2001), which is considered the gold standard. Their

designs have been driven by speed of administration, usually in the context of busy health care settings where time is of the essence. Alcohol screening questionnaires were initially tested and validated on populations of health care seekers and have since been used in other settings, such as criminal justice. Table 6.1 compares the most commonly used screening questionnaires and their salient features, and this table may be used to decide on the most appropriate measure.

Commonly used screening questionnaires
Alcohol Use Disorder Identification Test

The AUDIT comprises 10 questions addressing 4 areas: alcohol consumption, abnormal drinking behaviour and dependence, consumption and psychological effects and alcohol-related problems.

Score AUDIT as follows:

0–7 = low-risk drinking, including abstinence

8–15 = a medium level of alcohol problem ('hazardous' drinking)

16–19 = a high level of alcohol problem ('harmful' drinking)

20–40 = further evaluation for alcohol dependence required

Total scores of 8 or more indicate hazardous and harmful alcohol use as well as possible alcohol dependence (Babor et al., 2001).

Table 6.1 Summary of commonly used screening questionnaires

QUESTIONNAIRE ABBREVIATION	QUESTIONNAIRE TITLE	IDENTIFICATION	TARGET POPULATION/ SETTING	ADMINISTRATION TIME
AUDIT	Alcohol Use Disorders Identification Test	Hazardous harmful and dependent drinkers	Wide range of settings First choice in community setting	120 seconds
AUDIT-C[a]		Hazardous	Short form AUDIT	60 seconds
AUDIT-PC[a]		Hazardous Harmful	Short form AUDIT	60 seconds
FAST[a]	Fast Alcohol Screening Test	Hazardous Harmful	Various A&E	12 seconds
M-SASQ	Single Alcohol Screening Question	Hazardous Harmful	Various, including criminal justice	10 seconds
PAT	Paddington Alcohol Test	Hazardous Harmful	A&E	25 seconds
CAGE	CAGE	Dependent drinkers	Widespread use in clinical practice	60 seconds
T-ACE[b]	T-ACE	Hazardous Harmful	Antenatal settings	<120 seconds
TWEAK[b]	TWEAK	Hazardous Harmful	Antenatal settings General population (male and female)	<120 seconds

[a]Questionnaire based on items from AUDIT.
[b]Questionnaire based on items from CAGE.
Source: Alcohol Learning Centre (2012).

Alcohol Use Disorder Identification Test—Consumption

A revised version of AUDIT, the Alcohol Use Disorders Identification Test—Consumption (AUDIT-C), uses only the first three questions of AUDIT to screen for hazardous or harmful drinking and potential alcohol dependence.

http://www.alcohollearningcentre.org.uk/Topics/Browse/BriefAdvice/?parent=4444&child=4898.

Alcohol Use Disorder Identification Test—Primary Care

The Alcohol Use Disorder Identification Test—Primary Care (AUDIT-PC) provides an adapted Primary Care version of the full AUDIT.

http://www.alcohollearningcentre.org.uk/Topics/Browse/BriefAdvice/?parent=4444&child=4897.

FAST Alcohol Screening Test

The FAST Alcohol Screening Test (FAST) is a four-item screening test created from AUDIT. It was developed for busy clinical settings as a two-stage initial screening test that is quick to administer. More than half of patients are identified using only the first question.

http://www.alcohollearningcentre.org.uk/Topics/Browse/BriefAdvice/?parent=4444&child=4570.

Modified Single Alcohol Screening Question

The Modified Single Alcohol Screening Question (M-SASQ) is a one-question identification tool.

www.alcohollearningcentre.org.uk/Topics/Browse/BriefAdvice/?parent=. . . .

Paddington Alcohol Test 2011

The Paddington Alcohol Test (PAT) is an evolving pragmatic clinical tool, which is updated annually. It detects early stage alcohol misuse and seeks to maximise the link between Accident and Emergency department (A & E) attendance, alcohol issues and motivation by minimising the delay in referral to an alcohol counsellor.

http://www.alcohollearningcentre.org.uk/Topics/Browse/Hospitals/EmergencyMedicine/?parent=5168&child=5169.

Cutting down, Annoyance by criticism, Guilty feeling, and Eye-openers

The CAGE questions focus on Cutting down, Annoyance by criticism, Guilty feeling, and Eye-openers. The acronym 'CAGE' helps practitioners recall the questions. The CAGE questionnaire (Mayfield et al., 1974) is a four-item questionnaire that focuses on:

Cutting down on drinking

Annoyed by criticism

Guilty feeling

Eye-opener (early morning drink)

Responding positively to at least two of the questions indicates a need for further investigation and potential alcohol dependence.

http://www.ncbi.nlm.nih.gov/pubmed/6471323.

Take number of drinks, Annoyed, Cut down, Eye opener

T-ACE is a four-item questionnaire (Take number of drinks, Annoyed, Cut down, Eye opener) that is based on CAGE (Sokol et al., 1989). It is designed to identify risky drinking in women who are pregnant, and it varies from CAGE in that it asks a question about alcohol tolerance: 'How many drinks does it take to make you feel high?' More than two drinks indicates risk.

A total score of two or more indicates potential risk.

http://www.mhqp.org/guidelines/perinatalPDF/T-ACEScreeningTool.pdf.

Tolerance, Worried, Eye-opener, Amnesia, Kut down

Tolerance, Worried, Eye-opener, Amnesia, Kut down (TWEAK) is a five-item scale developed originally to screen for risky drinking during pregnancy. The questions focus on the following themes:

Tolerance

Worried

Eye-opener

Amnesia (blackouts)

K: cut down

Scoring TWEAK test

The maximum score is seven points; the first two questions count for two points each. If a woman responds that it takes three or more drinks to feel high (Tolerance), she scores two points.

A total score of two or more indicates harmful drinking and further evaluation is needed.

http://alcoholism.about.com/od/tests/a/tweak.htm.

There is a broad consensus among patients and health care professionals that a targeted, as opposed to universal, approach represents best practice and use of resources. Screening everyone could create more problems than it solves and may therefore diminish the impact of subsequent ABIs and consequent health benefits.

A wide range of screening tools, described above, can be used to identify hazardous and harmful drinking in health, criminal justice and other settings. Drinking behaviour can be screened routinely, the exception being those who directly seek assistance for an alcohol problem. If a screening test indicates hazardous or harmful drinking, a brief intervention can be offered. For higher scores, further assessment using AUDIT should be done in order to identify the nature of the alcohol consumption, pattern and consequences. In turn, this assessment would indicate the type of brief intervention required or that further assessment of drinking consequences needs to be explored via specialist intervention. This is best practice as recommended by Raistrick et al. (2006), the Scottish Intercollegiate Guidelines Network (SIGN, 2003) and the National Institute for Clinical Excellence (NICE, 2010a).

Alcohol brief interventions

Brief interventions, sometimes called *minimal interventions*, refer primarily to the duration of engagement by the health care or social care professional with the hazardous or harmful drinker. However, this does not necessarily mean that the process of change for that individual is fast or that the effort involved is minimal.

The number needed to treat (NNT) is central to ABI and is defined as the number of hazardous or harmful drinkers who need to receive an intervention for 1 drinker to reduce their consumption to within recommended limits. The NNT for ABIs is 8 (Moyer et al., 2002), whereas the NNT for smoking is 10, if nicotine replacement therapy is part of the intervention. Therefore, ABIs in a primary care setting are an effective use of resources.

A set of principles, informed by cognitive–behavioural and motivational methods, have emerged (Raistrick et al., 2006) which suggest that ABIs should

include six elements, based on the acronym FRAMES (see Box 6.1).

A wide range of methods of delivery of ABIs have been devised and tested, including brief counselling, written materials, self-help manuals and motivational interviewing (Robertson and Heather, 1998; Dunn et al., 2001; Carey et al., 2011); now, interactive interventions are available online (Box 6.2).

Box 6.1 FRAMES

*F*eedback: on risk and harm, from screening, assessment, or tests

*R*esponsibility: emphasis on personal responsibility for alcohol use and change

*A*dvice: clear, practical advice, and self-help material

*M*enu: options for change

*E*mpathy: non-judgemental and supportive attitudes

*S*elf-efficacy: increase an individual's belief in his or her ability to change

Source: Raistrick et al. (2006).

Box 6.2 ABI methods

- Leaflets
- Self-help manuals
- Brief counselling
- Brief motivational counselling
- Telephone contact and brief counselling
- Online interventions
- Self-monitoring

How brief is brief?

ABIs should be viewed as a continuum of increasing engagement. The duration of an ABI is likely to be restricted by organisational and workplace demands as opposed to identifying the most effective duration for an intervention. ABIs may differ in content and duration in an accident and emergency department, a general medical ward or a criminal justice setting.

Raistrick et al. (2006) outline two types of intervention:

Simple brief interventions consist of giving structured advice that takes no more than a few minutes to deliver, perhaps including giving the patient a leaflet on alcohol. This is sometimes described as *minimal intervention*. Poikolainen (1999) considered the distinction between very brief interventions (5–20 minutes) and 'extended' brief interventions that involved several contacts. Men and women benefited equally from very brief interventions, and only women benefited from extended brief interventions.

Extended brief interventions consist of structured therapies or psychosocial interventions that may take up to 30 minutes, possibly involving further and subsequent interventions. A 30-minute ABI script is outlined in Box 6.3.

The term *brief interventions* is also used in specialist alcohol treatment settings designed for people who are heavily dependent on alcohol and seek treatment, as opposed to those screened and identified opportunistically. In this context, *brief interventions* refer to interventions that may be used over a period of 4–5 hours, and their brevity is relative to lengthy standard treatment. Motivational Enhancement Therapy, one of the interventions tested in Project MATCH (Babor and Del Boca, 2003) and UKATT (UKATT, 2008) for dependent drinkers, was delivered in less than 4 hours; thus, it is sometimes referred to as a brief intervention.

Evidence for alcohol brief interventions

ABIs are commonly delivered opportunistically in a variety of health care settings. Since the early 1980s, a large body of research has been created on brief interventions, and a significant number of research reviews have been conducted. Their findings are broadly similar, in that they conclude that brief interventions are beneficial to the health of hazardous or harmful drinkers and to public health. Systematic reviews also demonstrate that ABIs should be restricted to those with problems of relatively low severity (Bien et al., 1993; Heather, 1994; Dunn et al., 2001; Moyer et al., 2002; Slattery et al., 2003; Babor et al., 2006). The Mesa Grande systematic review (Miller et al., 2003) ranks ABIs as the most effective, based on a substantial research track record of modest but positive outcomes, and this is reflected by the National Treatment Agency (England and Wales) recommendations on responding to

---

Box 6.3 The 15–30-minute motivational/ABI script

Background

The purpose of this script is to give you a template that will allow you to:

- raise the topic of and discuss alcohol consumption
- enable the client to indicate their level of concern about their drinking
- enable the client to consider what they might do about their situation

The wording of the script can be easily adapted to cover a wide range of health issues, all of which involve a motivational component as well as planned behaviour change as a means of reducing harm.

The script initially assumes that you have reported and explained health test findings or evidence of family concern or offending, with the intention of providing personalised feedback.

'You'll have seen/heard the test results for your health complaint (or seen your charge sheet or been made aware of the complaint)'.

'How do you feel about that?'

'Do you have any concerns relating to the test findings? Can you tell me about this?'

'OK, so how does that concern you?'

Recap the individual's statements as accurately as possible: 'So you're saying that your result concerns you because . . . And also you mentioned that you are concerned about . . .'.

'So do you think that something needs to change or that you need to make changes?'

'What needs to change? How could things be made better?'

'How do you think you'll go about making changes?'

'Can I summarise? Your drinking appears to be risky. You've said that you were concerned about your health and finances and were particularly worried because your mother drank heavily. Is that correct?'

'You also said that you thought cutting down might be a good idea. Can I give you an alcohol information leaflet, with some useful contacts, including my phone number?'

Practice makes perfect so try this with a friend.

---

alcohol problems in the UK (SIGN, 2003; Raistrick et al., 2006; Cobiac et al., 2009; NICE, 2010a). Despite evidence of ABI's effectiveness, the mechanisms of change are unclear. However, self-monitoring techniques in manuals and guidelines for reducing alcohol consumption are associated with improved outcomes (Michie et al., 2012).

! Thinking Point

Imagine you were using the script with each of the case studies in Box 6.4. Which of the three are you least likely to be successful with, and which of the three is more likely to respond positively to the ABI, and why?

Box 6.4 Case studies

Case #1: Brendan (age 43) consulted his GP for the first time in 10 years with the vague health complaints of feeling unwell, stomach upset, sleeplessness and depressed mood. The practice nurse conducted a screening procedure that indicated there was a problem with alcohol that might not respond to a brief intervention. The practice nurse suggested that Brendan conduct a fuller investigation of his drinking, with possible referral to a specialist treatment service for alcohol dependence. He drinks the same amount as his friends and is rather angry and bemused at the suggestion that he drinks too much.

Case #2: Elizabeth (age 23) is considering starting a family. In a routine health discussion, it emerged that her alcohol consumption was hazardous and might affect both her ability to conceive and the health of the foetus should she continue to drink at this level. She was keen to discuss this further and take home literature on alcohol information and cutting down consumption so she could discuss the issue with her partner.

Case #3: David (age 26) appeared in court following a binge drinking episode during which he assaulted one of his friends (though he had no recollection of the incident). He has a record of alcohol-related offences. As a condition of a probation order, he was mandated to participate in brief alcohol counselling. He is unhappy about this but has indicated to the alcohol worker and his probation officer that he will comply as he does not wish to be returned to court for non-compliance.

Screening and ABI in service settings

This section presents the available evidence on screening for alcohol consumption and problems opportunistically in a range of settings. This is followed by an evaluation of the effectiveness of ABIs in these settings. It should be noted that the outcomes will vary from one setting to the next even though the ABIs may be quite similar. Outcomes may relate to reductions in consumption, health or social problems, accidents, re-attendance at hospital or re-arrest, all of which reflect the main functions of the service setting.

Primary care

The majority of the population in the UK access health care via primary care services, including general practitioners. 'General practitioners and other primary health care staff should opportunistically identify hazardous and harmful drinkers and deliver a brief (10 minute) intervention', state the Scottish Intercollegiate Guidelines (SIGN, 2003). In an evaluation of the impact of strategies promoting screening and brief intervention by nursing professionals, Kaner et al. (2002) investigated three interventions: written guidelines (control group), outreach training and training with telephone-based support. The two experimental groups demonstrated higher levels of use in routine practice. Despite this, the control group was more accurate in their application of their intervention and made fewer errors. Overall, the balance of evidence suggests the use of written guidelines by nurses in primary care.

In a US study, more than 600 adults over age 55 were randomly assigned to receive a booklet on health behaviours (control group) or an intervention, which included personalised feedback, information on alcohol and ageing, a drink diary and telephone advice over a period of up to 8 weeks. At 12 months follow-up, there was no reduction in the proportion of heavy drinkers in the sample; however, there was evidence of a reduction in alcohol consumption (Moore et al., 2011).

An Australian study on the increasing mortality of liver disease among opioid-dependent people indicates a need to reduce long-term Hepatitis C virus (HCV) and other risks to the liver, including alcohol consumption. Cucciare and Weingardt (2011) propose ABIs as a first-line approach in addressing harmful levels of drinking in ageing opioid-dependent individuals with HCV. This is consistent with a Scottish study of recipients of methadone maintenance therapy, a substantial proportion of whom were HCV positive and drank harmfully; 20% had sought specialist alcohol treatment (O'Rawe, 2007).

Accident and emergency services

In a comparison study of the FAST (Hodgson et al., 2003), CAGE, and the PAT (Smith et al., 1996) in UK accident and emergency departments, all three were quicker to administer (<1 minute) than the full AUDIT (Babor et al., 2001; Hodgson et al., 2003). AUDIT is considered the gold standard, but it has been subject to alterations to shorten the administration time.

In an accident and emergency setting in the United States, brief interventions were evaluated as a routine component of trauma care (Gentilello et al., 1999). Those who screened positive were randomly allocated to a brief intervention or control group. At 12 months follow-up, the group who received the brief intervention had reduced their alcohol consumption significantly more than the control group. Those with mild to moderate alcohol problems were more likely to reduce their consumption. Following brief interventions, there was a 47% reduction in injuries requiring emergency or trauma centre admission and a 48% reduction in injuries requiring hospital admission. Researchers who conducted a similar study of a brief intervention based on the principles of motivational interviewing concluded that a brief motivational intervention for alcohol, plus a booster session, resulted in a reduction in subsequent trauma at 1 year follow-up of non-critically injured patients in a trauma centre whose alcohol consumption was hazardous or harmful (Mello et al., 2005). In the UK, Crawford et al. (2004) investigated the impact of a screening and brief intervention that had been incorporated into standard practice in an accident and emergency department. The experimental group received a leaflet and a 30-minute patient-centred discussion of their alcohol consumption with a health care worker, while the control group received only a leaflet. Significant reductions in consumption in the experimental group were evident at 6 and 12 months follow-up. As with other accident and emergency service studies, a reduction in service demand was observed.

A review of research on brief interventions in emergency and trauma services in the USA concluded that screening and brief interventions for alcohol-related problems were effective and that they should be incorporated into routine clinical practice. Researchers further report that clinicians in emergency services consider performing a brief intervention to be both feasible and acceptable in everyday practice, in spite of specific challenges such as time constraints and ethical and legal issues (D'Onofrio and Degutis, 2011).

General medical wards

A substantial proportion of patients in general medical wards may be hazardous or harmful drinkers. Raistrick et al.

(2006) recommend against the use of brief interventions in general medical wards because of inconclusive evidence of effectiveness. However, in a study conducted in general medical wards in Edinburgh, Chick et al. (1985) compared a 1-hour intervention by a nurse with a 'treatment as normal' control group, and both groups showed improvement (as might be expected of alcohol consumption at a time of ill health); however, the brief intervention group also demonstrated greater reductions in alcohol-related harm at follow-up.

Antenatal services

The risk to an unborn foetus from the mother's hazardous or harmful drinking makes identification of these patients an important health care function. Two screening instruments are commonly used, both of which are based on CAGE and take about 1 minute to administer:

T-ACE (Take number of drinks, Annoyed, Cut down, Eye-opener) (Sokol et al., 1989) and

TWEAK (Russell, 1994).

In an evaluation of screening questionnaires used in antenatal services T-ACE, TWEAK and AUDIT-C showed promise, while CAGE performed poorly (Burns et al., 2010). Additionally, TWEAK appears to be an efficient screening tool for men and women who are not pregnant, reflecting the broad relevance of the questions. These questionnaires and their scoring guides were discussed earlier in the chapter.

In a Swedish study, the AUDIT was used to examine the prevalence of hazardous or harmful alcohol consumption in pregnant women who were admitted for 1 year to an antenatal clinic in Stockholm. AUDIT scores were obtained for 1101 women for the year prior to pregnancy, and 17% reported AUDIT scores of 6 or higher, indicating hazardous or harmful alcohol consumption. There were few reports of alcohol dependence, but almost 50% of the women reported binge drinking at least once per month, and 6% reported binge drinking on every drinking occasion. One-third of the subjects (30%) continued regular alcohol use during pregnancy, and 6% reported drinking alcohol two to four times per month. AUDIT scores for the year prior to pregnancy and subject age, but not education level, predicted alcohol use during pregnancy. This screening test detected consumption during pregnancy in a manner which regular antenatal care did not; thus, Göransson et al. (2003) recommend it as part of routine antenatal care.

Chang et al. (2005) provide strong evidence in support of screening and ABIs in antenatal care settings. They suggest that as no safe level of alcohol use has been agreed on, it is useful to modify a woman's alcohol consumption early in her pregnancy and, in turn, reduce foetal risks. Chang's brief intervention studies demonstrated a greater likelihood of abstinence at follow-up and found that women with the highest levels of consumption made the greatest reductions. Furthermore, the effects of ABIs were enhanced by the involvement of a partner.

Offender services

A variety of connections between drinking and offending have been identified, and these are elaborated in Chapter 2. The screening questionnaires outlined above have been used to identify hazardous, harmful and dependent drinkers in a range of criminal justice settings: arrest-referral, probation services and prison.

A Home Office review of arrest-referral schemes in England was conducted to identify whether the benefits of reduced consumption following ABIs in health settings could result in a reduction in re-offending for those arrested for alcohol-related offences. Arrest-referral schemes have been a popular means of early intervention with offenders. Two major evaluations of pilot alcohol arrest-referral schemes carried out in England were designed to analyse the characteristics of those engaged in the services, establish whether ABIs could reduce offending, and identify any changes in alcohol consumption, health and wellbeing (Blakeborough and Richardson, 2012). Those over the age of 18 who had been arrested and were deemed to be under the influence of alcohol were targeted (excluding those arrested for drink driving offences), with a view to offering ABIs. The AUDIT questionnaire was used to evaluate individual arrestees' drinking, indicating that 35% were hazardous, 11% were harmful and 38% were dependent drinkers. The high proportion of dependent drinkers was unexpected, perhaps indicating the need for a referral route to specialist services. The researchers concluded that there was no strong evidence that ABIs following arrest reduce re-arrest though there was a weak indication of reduction in alcohol consumption. It is suggested that delivering ABIs to those in a custody suite is not an effective way to reduce offending. Insufficient screening was undertaken to identify those most likely to respond to ABIs; this is reflected in the service user statistic of 38% alcohol-dependent drinkers (AUDIT score 20+) who would benefit from more intensive assessment and intervention, including specialist treatment for alcohol problems. More than 50% of those arrested for alcohol-related offences had not been arrested in the previous 6 months, suggesting that those arrested during the night-time drinking hours were not prolific offenders: over one-third of arrests were for violent offences, and the rest were for petty alcohol-related offences (drunk and disorderly, criminal damage, public disorder), with the exception of drink driving arrests, which were 10% of the arrests in only one of the evaluations. Delivering ABIs in a custody setting is possible; however, good cooperation between custody staff and alcohol workers is required.

Of the three criminal justice settings, probation was found to be the most suitable for alcohol screening. A higher percentage of those approached took part: 81% in probation, 36% in prison, and 10% in police settings. Furthermore, participants in probation settings were positive about receiving interventions for their alcohol use (Coulton et al., 2012). In a study of alcohol screening and brief interventions in probation settings in England, FAST was judged to be a more efficient and effective screening tool than M-SASQ (McGovern et al., 2012). Three brief interventions of varying intensity were compared: an information leaflet (100% uptake), 5 minutes of brief advice (97% uptake) and a brief lifestyle counselling session of 20 minutes' duration (41% uptake). All interventions resulted in significant reductions in excessive alcohol consumption at 6 and 12 months follow-up, with a greater impact at 12 months. Consistent with a stepped-care approach, those scoring 8–15 on AUDIT benefited from simple feedback and an alcohol information leaflet, which was considered the most cost-effective intervention within the probation setting, while the benefits of the more intensive intervention were only apparent in those heavy drinkers scoring more than 16 on AUDIT. Barriers to implementation of ABIs in probation settings were related to workload pressures, and successful implementation was associated with management championing the approach and requiring additional specialist support in order to conduct both screenings and ABIs (McGovern et al., 2012).

In a Scottish prison study (MacAskill et al., 2011), AUDIT scores indicated that 73% of prisoners had an alcohol use disorder (8+) and 36% had scores indicating 'possible dependence' (20–40). Scores indicating 'possible dependence' were most apparent among 18–24 and 40–64-year-olds (40% and 56%, respectively), a finding confirmed using an altered version of CAGE (ISD, 2011). A high prevalence of alcohol use; varied problem behaviours; and links among drinking, crime and recidivism support the argument for more extensive provision of alcohol-focused interventions in prisons. The study concludes that initial screening and assessment should form the basis of a carefully targeted stepped-care approach ranging from ABIs to linking prisoners to community services (MacAskill et al., 2011). Unlike Coulton et al. (2012), there was no indication given of the acceptability of an alcohol intervention.

Within the criminal justice system, ABIs might form part of the already extensive range of services designed as alternatives to custody (arrest-referral, probation, community service) as well as part of the through-care and pre-liberation services provided within the prison system.

Educational institutions: Young people

A study conducted at inner London further education colleges compared a control group of 16–20-year-old students with a group who received a brief intervention; the focus was on influencing their use of drugs (including cannabis), alcohol and tobacco. The extended brief intervention (a 1-hour session of motivational interviewing) showed a reduction in levels of alcohol and cannabis use at 3 months, which almost disappeared after 12 months. There was also a reduction in use in the control group (McCambridge and Strang, 2004, 2005). In a Scottish study of further and higher education students, 65% of whom were binge drinkers (mean age 23 years), a 1-hour cognitive–behavioural educational session was offered. Subsequently, binge drinkers' positive attitudes toward binge drinking and their intention to binge drink shifted toward the beliefs held by non-binge drinkers. However, binge drinkers persisted in their belief that binge drinking was more prevalent among peers than did the non-binge drinkers (Marks and O'Connor, 2011).

Young people's alcohol consumption is characterised by binge drinking, and brief interventions may therefore be an important element in any strategy to reduce consumption and alcohol-related consequences. The evidence indicates that brief interventions have a positive impact on young people's drinking and drug use though the duration of impact may be limited compared to older hazardous and harmful drinkers identified opportunistically in health services, where the impact of ABIs appears more enduring. Educational establishments appear to be an appropriate setting for ABIs in the context of student health and welfare. While educational attainment may be affected by binge drinking, greater public concern is expressed for alcohol-related offending.

Family

The potential for brief interventions delivered in social and health care settings to target children and families and community-care clients is significant. Brief interventions were offered to people in the Midlands and South West England who were affected by the alcohol or drug use of a close family member. Relatives ($N = 143$) were randomly allocated to either a full or brief intervention, both of which were delivered by health care professionals. The purpose of the intervention was to focus on the needs of the family members in their own right, as opposed to directing the drinker into specialist services. The 'full' intervention consisted of up to five sessions, using a structured manual that focused on substance use, stress coping and support; in addition, the family member was given a self-help version of the intervention manual. The brief intervention consisted of one session, during which the content of the self-help manual was explained and the family member was encouraged to make use of the manual in their own time. Stress and coping measures at 12 weeks follow-up showed no difference between the two groups. Researchers concluded that a well-

constructed self-help manual delivered by a health care professional was likely to be as effective as several face-to-face contacts between health professionals and family members (Copello et al., 2009a,b). Furthermore, in interviews, clients reported (1) an increased awareness of the drinking relative's situation and that person's impact on the family, (2) a greater acknowledgement of the family members' own needs and rights, (3) an increased resolve to be assertive about plans and expectations, and (4) a general calming and reduction in physical and psychological symptoms of stress. The health professionals described their clients/subjects as happier, more confident, more assertive, less anxious, and/or depressed, and found that their clients were eating better and smoking less.

ABI barriers: The workforce

Despite clear evidence of ABI's effectiveness, efforts to encourage health professionals to incorporate screening and ABIs in their professional repertoire have met with limited success. As a result, a large amount of research literature has investigated the obstacles to implementation. Since the 1970s, research has confirmed the reluctance of nurses, doctors and social workers (other than those working in specialist addiction services) to deal with alcohol problems (Shaw et al., 1978; Kaner et al., 1999;

Watson et al., 2011). The key findings suggested that workers lacked:
- Role Adequacy: workers' perception that they have the knowledge and skills to work with problem drinkers
- Role Legitimacy: the perception that working with problem drinkers is part of their professional task
- Role Support: someone within the organisation who can provide advice, support, and guidance

It was noted that training events, designed to fill a gap in professional education, could increase health care and social workers' confidence in their knowledge and skills; however, their motivation to engage with problem drinkers remained low (Barrie, 1992). In comparing social workers with mental health nurses, Lightfoot and Orford (1986) concluded that social workers experienced a greater level of 'situational constraint' and, in turn, had less therapeutic commitment to working with problem drinkers. Organisational constraints consisted of time restrictions, lack of supervision or guidance and low priority for working with drinkers. Similarly, McGovern et al. (2012) noted that the workload priorities in busy probation services made the delivery of ABIs challenging without significant management support and specialist workers. In Scotland, attempts to influence situational constraints by training social workers and their managers resulted in greater role support and legitimacy, which was sustained, among those workers whose manager had received training (Duffy et al., 1998). However, these innovative post-professional qualification training ventures could never influence the curricula of the various professional training regimes, which appeared to (and still do) pay little attention to substance use issues. In a survey of social work students, 89% thought that the social work degree should include mandatory training on substance use problems, supporting the long-standing views of a special interest group of the British Association of Social Workers. In response, a representative of the Social Work Reform Board, charged with the profession's curriculum development, suggested that the topic must be weighed against many other pressing curriculum demands (Professional Social Work, 2011). Galvani and Forrester (2011) reviewed the evidence on social work and recovery for the Scottish government and concluded that formal social work education had failed to prepare social workers to work with substance users. Similar concerns were raised by Watson et al. (2011) with regard to nursing. It would appear that opportunities to focus more attention on substance use issues have been missed, especially during a period when both nursing and social work qualifications required students to study longer to obtain their degrees. The Scottish Government and the Convention of Scottish Local Authorities (COSLA) and Scottish Government (2010) identified the need to set learning priorities and competencies for all levels of the workforce on alcohol and drug issues, and they acknowledged the need for strategic leadership, both nationally and locally.

In a multicentre European study, Gilchrist et al. (2011) found that health professionals, nurses, doctors and social workers considered working with substance users to be of lower status than helping other patient groups. Lower status was also accorded to working with drug users as compared to drinkers. Substance users were seen to be less appealing, in particular to staff from primary care settings compared to staff from general psychiatry or specialist addiction services. Clearly, the workforce in primary care requires considerable support in order to be convinced that working with substance use issues, alcohol included, is a worthwhile and relevant activity. The root of such barriers to using ABIs lies in both the health and social policy arenas, where the relevance of ABIs to improving public health has not been supported by adequate resources and procedures. This is reflected in the professional education of those commonly in contact with hazardous and harmful drinkers (doctors, nurses and social workers), resulting in a sense of inadequacy and reluctance. Nilsen (2010) notes the professional barriers to implementation and suggests that further research in this area is likely to produce diminishing returns, presumably because the problems have been clearly delineated and now require a solution.

NHS Scotland appears to have addressed the stated barriers and implemented a scheme to integrate ABIs into routine health care practice, with a target of delivering 149,999 ABIs during the period 2008–2011; the target was exceeded within the deadline (Scottish Government, 2008a,b, 2011). At this stage, the impact of this approach has yet to be evaluated, and it remains to be seen whether ABIs will be integrated into routine practice beyond the project's duration. This policy intervention is in direct contradiction to Nilsen's (2010) suggestion that a 'top-down' approach to ABIs is not the best way forward. However, it's difficult to see how a programme designed to have an impact on an entire nation's health could feasibly be delivered other than by a centralised policy directive that is supported by appropriate resources and funding. See Box 6.5 for a list of resources and training opportunities.

Box 6.5 Resources and training opportunities

Structured information on alcohol brief interventions

IBA e-Learning Module & Alcohol Learning Centre
  http://www.alcohollearningcentre.org.uk/

SIPS Research Programme
  http://www.sips.iop.kcl.ac.uk/index.php

Continued

Box 6.5 Resources and training opportunities—cont'd

The Professional Development Award (PDA) in Brief Interventions for Substance Misuse at SCQF (Scottish Credit and Qualifications Framework) level 7 provides an SQA qualification for those working within the specialism of addictions and related services delivering brief interventions for substance misuse. It has been designed to provide a formal work-based qualification to improve professional practice and provide continuous professional development and progression to further higher and vocational qualifications (www.sqa.org.uk/sqa/48417.html (accessed 11/09/13)).

 Summary Points

(1) Identification of hazardous and harmful drinkers is the first step in offering ABIs. A number of screening questionnaires have been designed and tested, with both speed of administration and accuracy in mind. They are more effective and economic than traditional identification methods, such as biological markers, in most clinical or practice settings.

(2) ABIs represent a wide range of methods bound together by the brevity of professional input. There is evidence of a modest, but consistent, impact on consumption and consequences among hazardous and harmful drinkers (including binge drinkers), who are identified opportunistically, most commonly in health care settings.

(3) The potential for tackling alcohol issues at an earlier stage, implying lower levels of dependence and less severe and intractable problems, can make a substantial contribution to both individual and public health.

(4) ABIs are not recommended for those who are significantly dependent on alcohol but are effective ways to identify those who should be referred to specialist services.

(5) The evidence is strongest for ABIs, using a variety of methods both in health care settings (including accident and emergency, primary care, antenatal services) and in social work settings.

(6) Alcohol interventions appear more acceptable to those in probation settings within the criminal justice system.

(7) Barriers to the implementation of alcohol screening and ABIs in primary health care include lack of time and organisational priority.

(8) Inadequate professional training appears to contribute to the reluctance of professionals to engage with brief interventions and alcohol problems more generally.

Continued

(9) Continuing professional development, training and support can increase implementation and should be carefully adapted to meet the needs and attitudes of the workforce as well as the constraints of the service setting. The overall aim is to build role adequacy, legitimacy and support among staff in generic/non-alcohol specialist services so they will deliver ABIs.

(10) Given that much of the improvement in public health is a consequence of competent policy and funding, the future of ABIs rests with the enthusiasm of policymakers and their ability to overcome the obstacles and make the delivery of a public health benefit a reality.

(11) '[M]uch work remains to be done before BI is considered to be an integral part of mainstream preventive medicine and public health' —Nilsen (2010, p. 957).

Web pages and resources

http://www.scotland.gov.uk/About/Performance/scotPerforms/partnerstories/NHSScotlandperformance/alcoholbriefinterventions

The Scottish government's Web page on HEAT targets (Health improvement, Efficiency, Access, Treatment), with information on Scottish NHS Boards and how they are performing against the targets.

http://www.who.int/substance_abuse/activities/sbi/en/

This is the WHO page on screening and brief intervention for alcohol problems in primary health care. It contains access to WHO publications on the AUDIT, including a manual to help primary health care workers administer brief interventions.

http://www.alcoholconcern.org.uk/publications/factsheets/brief-interventions-factsheet

Provides access to a factsheet that looks at the five screening and brief intervention programmes operating in England, identifies common themes, such as the difficulties the programme operators have faced implementing the projects, and highlights pointers for success.

Further reading

Raistrick, D., Heather, N., Godfrey, C., 2006. Review of the Effectiveness of Treatment for Alcohol Problems. National Treatment Agency for Substance Misuse. NHS, London.
This document provides accessible information about the effectiveness of alcohol treatment to commissioners, managers and providers of alcohol treatment programmes.

Kaner, E., Dickinson, H., Beyer, F., Pienaar, E., Schlesinger, C., Campbell, F., Saunders, J., Burnand, B., Heather, N., 2009. The effectiveness of brief alcohol interventions in primary care settings: a systematic review. Drug Alcohol Rev. 28 (3), 301–323.
This review aims to assess the effectiveness of brief interventions in primary care and determine if outcomes differ between efficacy and effectiveness trials.

References

Abel, E.L., Sokol, R.J., 1986. Fetal alcohol syndrome is now leading cause of mental retardation. Lancet 2 (8517), 1222.

Advisory Council on the Misuse of Drugs, 2007. Hidden harm three years on: realities, challenges and opportunities. ACMD, Home Office, London.

Al-Anon UK and Eire. http://www.al-anonuk.org.uk/about/is-al-anon-for-you.html (accessed 3 March 2013).

Alati, R., Maloney, E., Hutchinson, D., Najam, J., Mattick, R., Bor, W., Williams, G., 2010. Do maternal parenting practices predict problematic patterns of adolescent alcohol consumption? Addiction 105 (5), 872–880.

Alcohol Concern, 2010a. Factsheet: information and statistical digest. Alcohol Concern, London.

Alcohol Concern, 2010b. Swept under the carpet: children affected by parental alcohol misuse. Alcohol Concern, London. http://www.alcoholconcern.org.uk/assets/files/Publications/Swept%20under%20the%20carpet.pdf (accessed 14 February 2013).

Alcohol Concern, 2013. Workplace alcohol solutions. Alcohol Concern, London. http://www.alcohollearningcentre.org.uk/eLearning/IBA/ (accessed 16 April 2014).

Alcohol Concern Cymru, 2010. A drinking nation? Wales and alcohol. Alcohol Concern, London.

Alcohol Concern Cymru, 2012. On the front line: alcohol and the armed forces. Alcohol Concern Cymru, Cardiff.

Alcohol Learning Centre, 2012. Identification and brief advice tools and techniques. http://www.alcohollearningcentre.org.uk/eLearning/IBA/ (accessed 16 April 2014).

Alcoholics Anonymous, 2013. 12 Steps. http://www.alcoholics-anonymous.org.uk/About-AA/The-12-Steps-of-AA (accessed 2 August 2013).

Anton, R., O'Malley, S., Ciraulo, D., Cisler, R., Couper, D., Donovan, D.M., COMBINE Study Research Group, 2006. Combined pharmacotherapies and behavioural interventions for alcohol dependence. The COMBINE study: a randomized controlled trial. JAMA 293, 2003–2017.

Babor, T., Del Boca, F. (Eds.), 2003. Treatment Matching in Alcoholism. Cambridge University Press, Cambridge.

Babor, T., Higgins-Biddle, J.C., Saunders, J.B., Monteiro, M.G., 2001. AUDIT: The Alcohol Use Disorders Identification Test – Guidelines for Use in Primary Care, second ed. World Health Organization, Geneva.

Babor, T., Caetano, R., Casswell, S., Edwards, G., Giesbrecht, N., Graham, K., Grube, J., Gruenwald, P., Hill, L., Holder, H., Homel, R., Osterberg, E., Rehm, J., Room, R., Rossow, I., 2003. Alcohol: No Ordinary Commodity: Research and Public Policy. Oxford University Press, Oxford.

Babor, T., Higgins-Biddle, J., Dauser, D., Burleson, J., Zarkin, G., Bray, J., 2006. Brief interventions for at-risk drinking: patient outcomes and cost-effectiveness in managed care organisations. Alcohol Alcohol. 41 (6), 624–631.

Banks, I., 2003. Raw Spirit: In Search of the Perfect Dram. Century, London.

Barrie, K., 1990. Helping in groups. In: Collins, S. (Ed.), Alcohol, Social Work and Helping. Routledge, London.

Barrie, K., 1992. Professional training. In: Plant, M., Ritson, B., Robertson, R. (Eds.), Alcohol and Drugs: The Scottish Experience. Edinburgh University Press, Edinburgh.

Barrie, K., 2012. Alcohol. Dunedin Academic Press, Edinburgh.

Beale, S., Sanderson, D., Kruger, J., Glanville, J., Duffy, S., 2009. The societal cost of alcohol misuse in Scotland in 2007. Research Findings No. 89/2009. Social Research. Scottish Government, Edinburgh.

Berglund, M., 2005. A better widget? Three lessons for improving addiction treatment from a meta-analytical study. Addiction 100, 742–750.

Best, D., Rome, A., Hanning, K., White, W., Gossop, M., Taylor, A., Perkins, A., 2010. Research for recovery: a review of the drugs evidence base. Scottish Government, Edinburgh.

Betty Ford Consensus Panel, 2007. What is recovery? A working definition from the Betty Ford Institute. J. Subst. Abuse Treat. 33, 221–228.

Bien, T., Miller, W., Tonigan, S., 1993. Brief interventions for alcohol problems: a review. Addiction 88 (3), 315–336.

Bischof, G., Rumpf, H., Hapke, U., Meyer, C., John, U., 2000. Maintenance factors of recovery from alcohol dependence in treated and untreated individuals. Alcohol. Clin. Exp. Res. 24, 1773–1777.

Bischof, G., Rumpf, H., Hapke, U., Meyer, C., John, U., 2003. Types of natural recovery from alcohol dependence: a cluster analysis approach. Addiction 98, 1737–1746.

Black, H., Gill, J., Chick, J., 2011. The price of a drink: levels of consumption and price paid per unit of alcohol by Edinburgh's ill drinkers with a comparison to wider alcohol sales in Scotland. Addiction 104, 4.

Blakeborough, L., Richardson, A., 2012. Summary of findings from two evaluations of Home Office Arrest referral pilot schemes. Research Report 60. Home Office, London.

Bodin, M., Strandberg, A., 2011. The Orebro prevention programme revisited: a cluster-randomized effectiveness trial of programme effects on youth drinking. Addiction 106, 9.

Booth, A., Meier, P., Stockwell, T., et al., 2008. Part A: systematic reviews. School of Health and Related Research, University of Sheffield, Sheffield.

Bottled Up. http://bottled-up.memberlodge.com (accessed 1 July 2013).

Braiden, G., 2011. Warning over alcohol bans on under 21s: SNP could face backlash from young people. Herald 1 June 2011.

Brennan, A., Purshouse, R., Rafia, R., Taylor, K., Meier, P., 2008. Independent review of alcohol pricing and promotion: part B results from the Sheffield Alcohol Policy Model. University of Sheffield, Sheffield.

British Crime Survey, 2011. Crime in England and Wales 2010 to 2011. Findings from the British Crime Survey and police recorded crime, second ed. Home Office, London. Crown Copyright. https://www.gov.uk/government/uploads/system/uploads/attachment_data/file/116417/hosb1011.pdf. (accessed 1 April 2014).

Bromley, C., Shelton, N., 2010. The Scottish Health Survey: UK Comparisons. Scottish Government, Edinburgh.

Bufe, C., 1998. Alcoholics Anonymous: Cult or Cure. See Sharp Press, Tucson.

Burns, E., Gray, R., Smith, L., 2010. Brief screening to identify problem drinking during pregnancy: a systematic review. Addiction 105, 601–614.

Carey, K., Carey, M., Henson, J., Maisto, S., DeMartini, K., 2011. Brief alcohol interventions for mandated college students: comparison of face to face counseling and computer delivered interventions. Addiction 106 (3), 528–537.

Casswell, S., Quan You, R., Huckle, T., 2011. Alcohol's harm to others: reduced well-being and health status for those with heavy drinkers in their lives. Addiction 106 (6), 1087–1094.

Chaloupka, F., 2009. Alcoholic beverage taxes, prices and drinking. Addiction 104, 191–192.

Chang, G., McNamara, T., Orav, E., et al., 2005. Brief intervention in prenatal alcohol use: a randomized trial. Obstet. Gynecol. 105, 991–998.

Chartered Institute of Personnel and Development, 2007. Managing drug and alcohol misuse at work. Survey Report 2007. CIPD.

Chick, J., Lloyd, G., Crombie, E., 1985. Counselling problem drinkers in medical wards: a controlled study. BMJ 290, 965–967.

Cobiac, L., Vos, T., Doran, C., Wallace, C., 2009. Cost-effectiveness of interventions to prevent alcohol-related disease and injury in Australia. Addiction 104 (10), 1646–1655.

Cochrane, R., Bal, S., 1990. Patterns of alcohol consumption in Sikh, Hindu and Muslim men in the West Midlands. Br. J. Addict. 85, 759–769.

Collins, E., Dickson, N., Eynon, C., et al., 2008. Drinking and driving 2007: prevalence, decision making and attitudes. Scottish Government Social Research, Edinburgh.

Commission of the European Communities, 2006. EU strategy to support Member States in reducing alcohol related harm – impact assessment report, Brussels. http://www.eumonitor.nl/9353000/1/j9vvik7m1c3gyxp/vi7jgt4c8oza.

Confederation of British Industry, 2011. Healthy returns? Absence and workplace health survey 2011. CBI.

Copello, A., Orford, J., 2002. Addiction and the family: is it time for services to take notice of the evidence? Addiction 97, 1361–1363.

Copello, A., Orford, J., Hodgson, R., Tober, G., 2009a. Social Behaviour and Network Therapy for Alcohol Problems. Routledge, East Sussex.

Copello, A., Templeton, L., Orford, J., Velleman, R., Patel, A., Moore, L., MacLeod, J., Godfrey, C., 2009b. The relative efficacy of two levels of a primary care intervention for family members affected by the addiction problem of a close relative: a randomised trial. Addiction 104, 49–58.

Coulton, S., Newbury-Birch, D., Cassidy, P., Dale, V., Deluca, P., Gilvarry, E., et al., 2012. Screening for alcohol use in criminal justice settings: an exploratory study. Alcohol Alcohol. 47, 423–427. http://dx.doi.org/10.1093/alcalc/ags048.

References

Crawford, M., Patton, R., Touquet, R., Drummond, C., Byford, S., et al., 2004. Screening and referral for brief intervention of alcohol-misusing patients in an emergency department. Lancet 364, 1334–1339.

Cucciare, M.A., Weingardt, K.R., 2011. Commentary on Gibson et al. (2011): Brief alcohol interventions in the context of treatment for hepatitis C. Addiction 106 (12), 2193–2194.

Davies, P., Walsh, D., 1983. Alcohol Problems and Alcohol Control in Europe. Croom Helm, London.

Department of Education, 2012. Children and young people: alcohol. http://www.education.gov.uk/childrenandyoungpeople/healthandwellbeing/substancemisuse/a0070043/alcohol (accessed 17 October 2012).

Department of Health, 1995. Sensible Drinking: report of an interdepartmental working group. DoH, London.

Department of Health, 1998. Independent inquiry into inequalities in health report. Stationary Office. https://www.gov.uk/government/publications/independent-inquiry (accessed 1 April 2014).

Department of Health, 2012a. The government's alcohol strategy. Crown Copyright. https://www.gov.uk/government/publications/alcohol-strategy (accessed 1 August 2013).

Department of Health, 2012b. Drug advice for schools: early intervention. http://www.education.gov.uk/aboutdfe/advice/f00202357/drug-advice-schools/intervention (accessed 17 October 2012).

Department of Health Social Services and Public Safety Northern Ireland, 2011. New strategic direction for alcohol and drugs: phase 2 2011–2016. A framework for reducing alcohol and drug related harm in Northern Ireland. DHSSPSNI, Belfast. www.dhsspsni.gov.uk (accessed 10 July 2012).

Di Clemente, C., 2006. Natural change and the troublesome use of substances: a life course perspective. In: Miller, W.R., Carroll, K.M. (Eds.), Rethinking Substance Abuse. Guilford Press, New York.

Di Clemente, C., Prochaska, J., 1998. Toward a comprehensive trans-theoretical model of change: stages of change in the addictive behaviours. In: Miller, W., Heather, N. (Eds.), Treating Addictive Behaviours: Processes of Change, second ed. Plenum, New York.

Donaldson, L., Rutter, P., 2011. Commentary on Black et al. (2011): Minimum pricing of alcohol – a solution whose time has come. Addiction 106 (4), 737–738.

D'Onofrio, G., Degutis, L., 2011. Screening and brief intervention in the emergency department. NIAAA. http://pubs.niaaa.nih.gov/publications/arh28-2/63-72.pdf (accessed 16 April 2014).

Drummond, C., Oyefeso, A., Phillips, T., Cheeta, S., et al., 2005. Alcohol Needs Assessment Research Project (ANARP). The 2004 ANARP for England. Department of Health, London.

Drummond, C., DeLuca, P., Oyefeso, A., Rome, A., et al., 2009. Scottish Alcohol Needs Assessment. Institute of Psychiatry, King's College, London.

Duffy, J., 1992. Scottish licensing reforms. In: Plant, M., Ritson, B., Robertson, R. (Eds.), Alcohol and Drugs: The Scottish Experience. Edinburgh University Press, Edinburgh.

Duffy, T., Holttum, S., Keegan, M., 1998. An investigation of the impact of training on social workers and their managers. Alcoholism 34, 93–104.

Dunbar, J., 1992. Drink and driving. In: Plant, M., Ritson, B., Robertson, R. (Eds.), Alcohol and Drugs: The Scottish Experience. Edinburgh University Press, Edinburgh.

Dunn, C., Deroo, L., Rivara, F., 2001. The use of brief interventions adapted from motivational interviewing across behavioural domains: a systematic review. Addiction 96 (12), 1725–1742.

DVLA. https://www.gov.uk/current-medical-guidelines-dvla-guidance-for-professionals-conditions-a-to-c (accessed 2 April 2014).

Eadie, D., MacAskill, S., Brooks, O., Helm, D., Forsyth, A., Punch, S., 2010. Pre-teen learning about alcohol: drinking and family contexts. Joseph Rowntree Foundation. www.jrf.org.uk.

E-cyclopedia 141 Words for Drunk. http://news.bbc.co.uk/1/hi/uk/1883481.stm (accessed 14 March 2014).

Edwards, G., 2000. Editorial note: natural recovery is the only recovery. Addiction 95, 747.

Effiong, K., Osinowo, A., Pring, A., 2012. Deaths from liver disease: implications for end of life care in England. National End of Life Care Intelligence Network. NHS. Crown Copyright. www.endoflifecare-intelligence.org.uk (accessed 10 July 2012).

Erskine, S., Maheswaran, R., Pearson, T., Gleeson, D., 2010. Socioeconomic deprivation, urban-rural location and alcohol-related mortality in England and Wales. BMC Public Health 10, 99. http://www.biomedcentral.com/1471-2458/10/99/ (accessed 13 August 2012).

European Alcohol and Health Forum, 2011. Alcohol, work and productivity: scientific opinion of the science group of the European alcohol and health forum. EU science_02_en.pdf.

Fazel, S., Bains, P., Doll, H., 2006. Substance abuse and dependence in prisoners: a systematic review. Addiction 101, 181–191.

Fear, N., Iversen, A., Meltzer, H., et al., 2007. Patterns of drinking in the UK armed forces. Addiction 102, 1749–1759.

Fernandez-Hermida, J., Calafat, A., Becona, E., Tsertsvadze, A., Foxcroft, D., 2012. Assessment of generalizability, applicability and predictability (GAP) for evaluating external validity in studies of universal family-based prevention of alcohol misuse in young people: systematic methodological review of randomized controlled trials. Addiction 107, 9.

Fiorentine, R., 1999. After drug treatment: are 12 step programs effective in maintaining abstinence. Am. J. Drug Alcohol Abuse 25 (1), 93–116.

Fitzpatrick, R., Thorne, L., 2010. A label for exclusion: support for alcohol-misusing offenders. Centre for Mental Health, London.

Forrester, D., 2000. Parental substance misuse and child protection in a British sample. Child Abuse Rev. 9 (4), 235–246.

Foxcroft, D., Tsertsvadze, A., 2011. Universal alcohol misuse prevention programmes for children and adolescents. Cochrane Review, Wiley.

Foxcroft, D., Ireland, D., Lowe, G., Breen, R., 2002. Primary prevention for alcohol misuse in young people. Cochrane Database Syst. Rev. (3), CD003024. http://dx.doi.org/10.1002/14651858.CD003024.

Galvani, S., 2010. Grasping the nettle: alcohol and domestic violence. Factsheet. Alcohol Concern, London. www.alcoholconcern.org.uk/publications/factsheets/grasping-the-nettle.

Galvani, S., Forrester, D., 2011. Social work services and recovery from substance misuse: a review of the evidence. In: Scottish Government Social Research. Crown Copyright.

Gartner, A., 2009. Alcohol and health: a profile of alcohol and health in Wales. Wales Centre for Health, Cardiff. http://www.wales.nhs.uk/sitesplus/888/news/14758 (accessed 16 April 2014).

Giesbrecht, N., Cukier, S., Steeves, D., 2010. Collateral damage from alcohol: implications of "second hand effects of drinking" for populations and health priorities. Addiction 105, 1323–1325.

Gentilello, L., Rivara, F., Donovan, D., Jurkovich, G., Daranciang, E., Dunn, C., Villaceces, A., Copass, M., Ries, R., 1999. Alcohol interventions in a trauma center as a means of reducing the risk of injury recurrence. Ann. Surg. 230 (4), 473.

Gibson, A., Randall, D., Degenhart, L., 2011. The increasing mortality burden of liver disease among opioid dependent people: cohort study. Addiction 106, 12.

Gilchrist, E., Johnson, R., Takriti, R., Weston, S., et al., 2003. Domestic violence offenders: characteristics and offending related needs. Findings 217 Home Office. Crown Copyright.

Gilchrist, G., Moskalewicz, J., Slezakova, S., Okruhlica, L., Torrens, M., Vajd, R., Baldacchino, A., 2011. Staff regard towards working with substance users: a European multi-centre study. Addiction 106 (6), 114–125.

Gmel, G., Kuntsche, E., Rehm, J., 2011. Risky single-occasion drinking: bingeing is not bingeing. Addiction 106 (6), 1037–1045.

Göransson, M., Magnusson, A., Bergman, H., Rydberg, U., Markus, H., 2003. Fetus at risk: prevalence of alcohol consumption during pregnancy estimated with a simple screening method in Swedish antenatal clinics. Addiction 98 (11), 1513–1520.

Gossop, M., Moos, R., 2008. Substance misuse among older adults: a neglected but treatable problem. Addiction 103, 347–348.

Gossop, M., Harris, J., Best, D., Man, L.-H., et al., 2003. Is attendance at Alcoholics Anonymous meetings after in-patient treatment related to improved outcomes? A 6-month follow-up study. Alcohol Alcohol. 38 (5), 421–426.

Gossop, M., Stewart, D., Marsden, J., 2008. Attendance at Narcotics Anonymous and Alcoholics Anonymous meetings, frequency of attendance and substance use outcomes after residential treatment for drug dependence: a 5 year follow up study. Addiction 103 (1), 119–125.

Granfield, R., Cloud, W., 1999. Coming Clean: Overcoming Addiction Without Treatment. New York University Press, New York.

Gray, L., 2007. Comparisons of health-related-behaviours and health measures between Glasgow and the rest of Scotland. Glasgow Centre for Population Health, Glasgow. http://www.gcph.co.uk/assets/0000/0384/GCPH_briefing_paper_FS_7_web.pdf (accessed 16 April 2014).

Green, C., Paniagua, M., 2013. Play hard, shirk hard: the effect of bar hours regulation on worker absence. University of Lancaster. www.lancs.ac.uk/staff/greencp/papers/PlayHardShirkHard.pdf (accessed 1 August 2013).

References

Griesbach, D., Lardner, C., Russell, P., 2009. Managing the needs of drunk and incapable people in Scotland: a literature review and needs assessment. Scottish Government Social Research.

Hanlon, P., Walsh, D., Whyte, B., 2006. Let Glasgow flourish. Glasgow Centre for Population Health, Glasgow.www.scotland.gov.uk/Publications/2010/11/10110338/19.

Harbin, F., Murphy, M. (Eds.), 2000. Substance Misuse and Child Care: How to Understand, Assist and Intervene When Drugs Affect Parenting. Russell House Publishing, London.

Harkins, C., Poley, D., 2011. Making alcohol policy: increasing consumption or reducing harm. Alcohol Alert 1, 20–22.

Harris, J., et al., 2003. Prior Alcoholics Anonymous (AA) affiliation and the acceptability of the twelve steps to patients entering UK statutory addiction treatment. J. Stud. Alcohol 64, 257–261.

Health and Safety Executive, 2002. Work environment, alcohol consumption and ill-health: The Whitehall 11 Study. HSE, London. http://www.hse.gov.uk/research/crr_pdf/2002/crr02422.pdf.

Health and Safety Executive, 2011. Don't mix it. A guide for employers on alcohol at work. HSE. www.hse.gov.uk/pubns/indg240.pdf (accessed 13 April 2013).

Health Scotland, 2006. Alcohol and Ageing: Is Alcohol a Major Threat to Healthy Ageing for the Baby Boomers? A Report by the Alcohol and Ageing Working Group. NHS Scotland, Edinburgh.

Heath, D., 2000. Drinking Occasions: Comparative Perspectives on Alcohol and Culture. Brunner-Routledge, London.

Heather, N., 1994. Interpreting the evidence on brief interventions for excessive drinkers: the need for caution. Alcohol Alcohol. 30 (3), 287–296.

Her Majesty's Government, 2012. The government's alcohol strategy. CM8336. HM Government. The Stationery Office, London. AlcoholStrategy@homeoffice.gsi.gov.uk (accessed 10 July 2012).

Hester, M., 2009. Who does what to whom? Gender and domestic violence perpetrators. University of Bristol, Bristol. http://www.bris.ac.uk/sps/research/projects/reports/2009/rj4843/whodoeswhat.pdf (accessed 16 April 2014).

Hillier, D., Fewell, F., Cann, W., Shepard, V., 2005. Wellness at work: enhancing the quality of our working lives. Int. Rev. Psychiatry 17 (5), 419–431.

HIV Scotland, 2012. HIV & alcohol: for people living with, or at risk, of HIV. HIV Scotland, Edinburgh.www.hivscotland.com.

HM Parliament, 2010. Alcohol Health Committee. The impact of alcohol on health, the NHS and society. http://www.publications.parliament.uk/pa/cm200910/cmselect/cmhealth/151/15107.htm (accessed 16 April 2014).

Hodgson, R., John, B., Abbasi, T., Hodgson, R., et al., 2003. Fast screening for alcohol misuse. Addict. Behav. 28, 1453–1463.

Holder, H., 2007. What we learn from a reduction in the retail alcohol prices: lessons from Finland. Addiction 102, 346–347.

Holder, H., 2010. Prevention programmes in the 21st century: what we do not discuss in public. Addiction 105, 578–581.

Homel, R., McIlwain, G., Carvolth, R., 2004. Creating safer drinking environments. In: Heather, N., Stockwell, T. (Eds.), The Essential Handbook of Treatment and Prevention of Alcohol Problems. Wiley & Sons, England.

Home Office, 2004. Guidance for local partnerships on alcohol related crime and disorder data. Development and Practice Report 6. Home Office, London.

Home Office, 2006. Violent Crime Reduction Act (2006). Home Office, London.

Home Office, 2011. Police Reform and Social Responsibility Act (2011). Home Office, London.

House of Commons Health Committee, 2010. Alcohol, vol. 1. House of Commons, Stationery Office, London.

House of Commons Select Committee, 2012. Alcohol guidelines – Science and Technology Committee Report. House of Commons, London.

Humphreys, K., Moos, R., 1996. Reduced substance abuse related health care costs among voluntary participants of AA. Am. Psychiatr. Assoc. 47, 709–713.

Humphreys, K., Moos, R., Finney, J., 1995. Two pathways out of drinking problems without professional treatment. Addict. Behav. 20 (4), 427–441.

Independent Inquiry into Drug Testing at Work, 2004. Drug testing in the workplace. Joseph Rowntree Foundation. www.jrf.org.uk.

Information Services Division, 2011. Alcohol Statistics Scotland 2011. NHS National Services Scotland. Common services/Crown Copyright.

Jenkins, R., Lewis, P., Bebbington, T., et al., 1997. The national psychiatric morbidity surveys of Great Britain – initial findings from the household survey. Psychol. Med. 27, 775–789.

Jones, L., Bellis, M., Dedman, D., Sumnall, H., Tocque, K., 2008. Alcohol attributable fractions for England: alcohol-attributable mortality and hospital admissions. John Moores University, North West Public Health Observatory, Liverpool.

Kaner, E., Heather, N., McAvoy, B., Lock, C., Gilvarry, E., 1999. Intervention for excessive alcohol consumption in primary health care: attitudes and practices of English general practitioners. Alcohol Alcohol. 34, 559–566.

Kaner, E., Locke, C., Heather, N., McNamee, P., Bond, S., 2002. Promoting brief alcohol intervention by nurses in primary care: a cluster randomised controlled trial. Patient Educ. Couns. 51 (3), 277–284.

Kaner, E., Dickinson, H., Beyer, F., Pienaar, E., Schlesinger, C., Campbell, F., Saunders, J., Burnand, B., Heather, N., 2009. The effectiveness of brief alcohol intervention in primary care settings: a systematic review. Drug Alcohol Rev. 28, 301–323.

Kaskutas, L., Ammon, L., Delucchi, K., Room, R., Bond, J., Weisner, C., 2005. Alcoholics anonymous careers: patterns of AA involvement five years after treatment entry. Alcoholism 29 (11), 1983–1990.

Kendell, R.E., de Roumanie, M., Ritson, E.B., 1983. Influence of an increase in excise duty on alcohol consumption and its adverse effects. Br. Med. J. 287, 809–811.

Keogh, P., et al., 2009. Wasted Opportunities. Sigma, England.www.sigmaresearch.org.uk/files/report2009c.pdf.

Klinger, E., Cox, M., 2004. Motivation and the theory of current concerns. In: Cox, M., Klinger, E. (Eds.), Handbook of Motivational Counselling: Concepts, Approaches and Assessment. Wiley, Cichester.

Klingemann, H., 2004. Natural recovery from alcohol problems. In: Heather, N., Stockwell, T. (Eds.), The Essential Handbook of Treatment and Prevention of Alcohol Problems. John Wiley & Sons, England.

Koski, A., Siren, R., Vuori, E., Poikolainen, K., 2007. Alcohol tax cuts and increase in alcohol-positive sudden deaths – a time-series intervention analysis. Addiction 102, 362–368.

Koutsakis, N., Stattin, H., Kerr, M., 2008. Reducing youth alcohol drinking through a parent-targeted intervention: the Orebro Prevention Program. Addiction 103, 1629–1637.

Kypri, K., Jones, C., McElduff, P., Barker, D., 2010. Effects of restricting pub closing times on night-time assaults in an Australian city. Addiction 106, 303–310.

Laslett, A., Room, R., Ferris, J., Wilkinson, C., et al., 2011. Surveying the range and magnitude of alcohol's harm to others in Australia. Addiction 106, 1603–1611.

Laslett, A., Room, R., Deitze, P., Ferris, J., 2012. Alcohol's involvement in recurrent child abuse and neglect cases. Addiction 107, 1786–1793.

Laudet, A., White, W., 2008. Recovery capital as prospective predictor of sustained recovery, life satisfaction, and stress among former poly-substance users. Subst. Use Misuse 43, 27–54.

Leask, D., 2010. Murder in private. Sunday Herald, 14 November 2010, Glasgow.

Leonard, K., 2011. Commentary on Livingston (2011). Addiction 106 (5), 926–928.

Lightfoot, P., Orford, J., 1986. Helping agents' attitudes towards alcohol related problems: situations vacant? A test and elaboration of a model. Br. J. Addict. 81 (6), 749–756.

Ling, J., Smith, K., Wilson, G., et al., 2012. The 'other' in patterns of drinking: a qualitative study of attitudes towards alcohol use among professional, managerial and clerical workers. BMC Public Health 12, 892. http://www.biomedcentral.com/1471-2458/12/892.

Livingston, M., 2011. A longitudinal analysis of alcohol outlet density and domestic violence. Addiction 106 (5), 919–925.

Lopez-Quintero, C., Hasin, D., de Los Cobos, P., Pines, A., Wang, S., Grant, B., Blanco, C., 2011. Probability and predictors of remission from lifetime nicotine, alcohol, cannabis and cocaine dependence: results from the National Epidemiologic Survey on Alcohol and Related Conditions. Addiction 106 (3), 657–669.

MacAskill, S., Parkes, T., Brooks, O., Graham, L., McAuley, A., Brown, A., 2011. Assessment of alcohol problems using AUDIT in a prison setting: more than an 'aye or no' question. BMC Public Health 11, 865. http://www.biomedcentral.com/content/pdf/1471-2458-11-865.pdf (accessed 16 April 2014).

MacGregor, A., Sharp, C., Mabelis, J., Corbett, J., 2013. An evaluation of the implementation of, and compliance with, the objectives of the Licensing (Scotland) Act 2005. Final Report ScotCen Social Research NHS Health Scotland. Edinburgh. http://www.healthscotland.com/documents/21321.aspx (accessed 17 April 2014).

References

Maclean, S., 2012. A qualitative investigation of nursing staff and physicians' knowledge and experience of Wernicke's Encephalopathy within an accident and emergency department. MSc Dissertation, University of the West of Scotland, Paisley.

Maisel, M., Blodgett, J., Wilbourne, P., Humphreys, K., Finney, J., 2013. Meta-analysis of naltrexone and acamprosate for treating alcohol use disorders: when are these medications most helpful? Addiction 108, 275–293.

Makela, P., Osterberg, E., 2009. Weakening of one more alcohol control pillar: a review of the effects of the alcohol tax cuts in Finland in 2004. Addiction 104, 554–563.

Marks, D., 2012. Qualification in Health Psychology (Stage 2) Portfolio of Competence. British Psychological Society, Leicester.

Marks, D., O'Connor, R., 2011. What influences binge drinking in students, and how can we intervene? Emotions 2011: Fifth International Conference on The (Non) Expression of Emotions in Health and Disease, Tilburg, the Netherlands (Oral Presentation).

Mayfield, D., McLeod, G., Hall, P., 1974. The CAGE questionnaire: validation of a new alcoholism screening instrument. Am. J. Psychiatry 131, 1121–1123.

McCambridge, J., Strang, J., 2004. The efficacy of a single-session motivational interviewing in reducing drug consumption and perceptions of drug related risk among young people: results from a multi-site cluster. Addiction 99, 39–52.

McCambridge, J., Strang, J., 2005. Deterioration over time in effect of motivational interviewing in reducing drug consumption and related risk among young people. Addiction 100, 470–478.

McCambridge, J., Hawkins, B., Holden, C., 2013. Industry use of evidence to influence alcohol policy: a case study of submissions to the 2008 Scottish government consultation. PLoS Med. 10 (4), e1001431. http://dx.doi.org/10.1371/journal.pmed.1001431, Published online April 23 2013.

McCartney, G., Collins, C., Walsh, D., Batty, D., 2011. Accounting for Scotland's excess mortality: towards a synthesis. Glasgow Centre for Population Health, Glasgow. http://www.scotpho.org.uk/comparative-health/excess-mortality-in-scotland-and-glasgow (accessed 16 April 2014).

McCready, B., 2006. Family and other close relationships. In: Miller, W., Carroll, K. (Eds.), Rethinking Substance Abuse: What the Science Shows, and What We Should Do About It. Guilford Press, New York, pp. 166–181.

McGovern, R., Newbury-Birch, D., Deluca, P., Drummond, C., 2012. Alcohol screening and brief intervention. SPIS CJS Factsheet. Institute of Psychiatry, King's College, London.

McMahon, J., Lewis, I., 2010. Bottled Up: How to Survive Living with a Problem Drinker. Lion Hudson, Oxford.

Measham, F., 2004. The decline of ecstasy, the rise of 'binge' drinking and the persistence of pleasure. Probat. J. 51 (4), 309–362.

Meier, P., Purshouse, R., Brennan, A., 2010. Policy options for alcohol price regulation: the importance of modelling population heterogeneity. Addiction 105, 383–393.

Mello, M., Nirenberg, T., Longabaugh, R., Woolard, R., Minugh, A., Becker, B., Baird, J., Stein, L., 2005. Emergency department brief motivational interventions for alcohol with motor vehicle crash patients. Ann. Emerg. Med. 45 (6), 620–625.

Meyers, R., Miller, W. (Eds.), 2001. A Community Reinforcement Approach to Addiction Treatment (International Research Monographs in the Addictions). Cambridge University Press, Cambridge.

Meyers, R., Miller, W., Smith, J., 2001. Community reinforcement and family training. In: Meyers, R., Miller, W. (Eds.), A Community Reinforcement Approach to Addiction Treatment (International Research Monographs in the Addictions). Cambridge University Press, Cambridge.

Michie, S., Whittington, C., Hamoudi, Z., Zarni, F., Tober, G., West, R., 2012. Identification of behaviour change techniques to reduce excessive alcohol consumption. Addiction 107, 8.

Midford, R., 2010. Drug prevention programmes for young people: where have we been and where should we be going? Addiction 105 (10), 1688–1695.

Miller, W., Wilbourne, P., Hettema, J., 2003. What works? A summary of alcohol treatment outcome research. In: Hester, R., Miller, W. (Eds.), Handbook of Alcoholism Treatment Approaches: Effective Alternatives. Allyn and Bacon, Boston.

Ministry of Defence, 2010. Shedding light on mental health in the forces. https://www.gov.uk/government/news/shedding-light-on-mental-health-in-the-forces (accessed 16 April 2014).

Ministry of Justice, 2012. LASPO amendments – alcohol abstinence and monitoring requirement. http://www.justice.gov.uk/downloads/legislation/bills-acts/legal-aid-sentencing/laspo-sobriety-ia.pdf (accessed 16 April 2014).

Moneysupermarket, 2012. Drink driving convictions. http://www.moneysupermarket.com/car-insurance/monitor-drink-driving-convictions/.

Moore, A., Blow, F., Hoffing, M., Welgreen, S., Davis, J., et al., 2011. Primary care based intervention to reduce at-risk drinking in older adults: a randomised controlled trial. Addiction 106, 111–120.

Moos, R., 2008. Active ingredients of substance use-focused self-help groups. Addiction 103 (3), 387–396.

Moyer, A., Finney, J., Swearingen, C., Vergun, P., 2002. Brief interventions for alcohol problems: a meta-analytic review of controlled investigations in treatment seeking and non-treatment-seeking populations. Addiction 97 (3), 279–292.

Muller, S., Piontek, D., Pabst, A., Baumeister, A., Kraus, L., 2010. Changes in alcohol consumption after the introduction of the alcopops tax in Germany. Addiction 105, 1205–1213.

Myers, R., Miller, W., Smith, E., 2001. Community reinforcement and family training (CRAFT). In: Myers, R., Miller, W. (Eds.), A Community Reinforcement Approach to Addiction Treatment. Cambridge University Press, Cambridge.

NHS Information Centre, 2010. Statistics on alcohol: England 2010. Health and Social Care Information Centre.

NHS Quality Improvement Scotland, 2005. Clinical Indicators 2005. NHS Scotland. www.indicators.scot.nhs.uk/Reports/2005_Clinical_Indicators_Report.pdf (accessed 16 April 2014).

NHS Scotland, 2009. Alcofacts: a guide to responsible drinking. Health Scotland, Edinburgh. www.healthscotland.com/documents/3269.aspx (accessed 16 April 2014).

National Institute for Clinical Excellence, 2007. Interventions in schools to prevent and reduce alcohol use among children and young people. NICE Public Health Guidance 7. NHS. www.nice.org.uk.

National Institute for Clinical Excellence, 2010a. Alcohol-use disorders: preventing the development of hazardous and harmful drinking. NICE Public Health Guidance 24. NHS. www.nice.org.uk.

National Institute for Clinical Excellence, 2010b. Alcohol-use disorders: diagnosis and clinical management of alcohol related physical complications. NICE Clinical Guidance 100. NHS. www.nice.org.uk.

National Institute for Clinical Excellence, 2011. Alcohol dependence and harmful alcohol use: NICE guidance CG115. NHS. www.nice.org.uk.

Neighbors, C., Brown, G., Dibello, A., Rodriguez, L., Foster, D., 2013. Reliance on God, prayer, and religion reduces influence of perceived norms on drinking. J. Stud. Alcohol Drugs 74, 361–368.

Niccols, A., Milligan, K., Sword, W., et al., 2012. Integrated programs for mothers with substance abuse issues: a systematic review of studies reporting on parenting outcomes. Harm Reduct. J. 9, 14. http://dx.doi.org/10.1186/1477-7517-9-14.

Nicholson Report, 2003. Review of Liquor Licensing Law in Scotland. Scottish Executive. Crown Copyright.

Nilsen, P., 2010. Brief alcohol intervention – where to from here? Challenges remain for research and practice. Addiction 105, 954–959.

Office for National Statistics, 2011. Smoking and drinking among adults, 2009: a report of the 2009 General Lifestyle Survey. ONS, Newport. http://www.ons.gov.uk/ons/rel/ghs/general-lifestyle-survey/2009-report/index.html (accessed 16 April 2014).

O'Malley, S., Kosten, T., 2006. Pharmacotherapy of addictive disorders. In: Miller, W., Carroll, K. (Eds.), Rethinking Substance Abuse: What the Science Shows, and What We Should Do About It. Guilford Press, New York.

O'Rawe, S., 2007. Investigating levels of problem drinking among those on methadone maintenance programmes: implications for individuals and services. MSc Thesis, University of the West of Scotland, Paisley.

Orford, J., 2001. Excessive Appetites: A Psychological View of Addictions, second ed. Wiley, Chichester.

Orford, J., 2008. Asking the right questions in the right way: the need for a shift in research on psychological treatments for addiction. Addiction 103 (6), 875–885.

Orford, J., Edwards, G., 1977. Alcoholism. Maudsley Monographs 26. Oxford University Press, Oxford.

Orford, J., Natera, G., Mora, J., Tiburcio, M., Copello, A., Velleman, R., 2005. Coping with Alcohol and Drug Problems. The Experience of Family Members in Three Contrasting Cultures. Routledge, London.

Ouimette, P., Moos, R., Finney, J., 1998. Influence of outpatient treatment and 12-step group involvement on one-year substance abuse treatment outcomes. J. Stud. Alcohol 59, 513–522.

Paljarva, T., Koskenvuo, M., Poikolainen, K., et al., 2009. Binge drinking and depressive symptoms: a 5 year population based cohort study. Addiction 104, 7.

Parsons, J., et al., 2004. Alcohol use and stigmatized sexual practices of HIV seropositive gay and bisexual men. Addict. Behav. 29, 1045–1051.

References

Paton, A., 2005. Alcohol in the body. Br. Med. J. 330, 85–87.

Percy, A., Wilson, J., McCartan, C., McCrystal, P., 2011. Teenage drinking cultures. Joseph Rowntree Foundation. www.jrf.org.uk.

Pidd, K., Boeckmann, R., Morris, M., 2006. Adolescents in transition: the role of workplace alcohol and other drug policies as a prevention strategy. Drug Educ. Policy Prev. 13 (4), 353–365.

Poikolainen, K., 1999. Effectiveness of brief interventions to reduce alcohol intake in primary health care populations: a meta-analysis. Prev. Med. 28 (5), 503–509.

Powis, B., Gossop, M., Bury, C., Payne, K., Griffiths, P., 2000. Drug using mothers: social psychological and substance use problems of women opiate users with children. Drug Alcohol Rev. 19 (2), 171–180.

Prime Minister's Strategy Office, 2004. Alcohol Harm Reduction Strategy for England. Cabinet Office, London.

Prison Reform Trust, 2004. Alcohol and re-offending – who cares? Prison Reform Trust. http://www.prisonreformtrust.org.uk/Portals/0/Documents/Alcohol%20briefing.pdf.

Prochaska, J., Di Clemente, C., 1983. Stages and processes of self-change of smoking: toward an integrative model of change. J. Consult. Clin. Psychol. 51, 390–395.

Professional Social Work, 2011. Social workers want more drugs and alcohol training. British Association of Social Workers, Birmingham.

Raistrick, D., Hodgson, R., Ritson, B. (Eds.), 1999. Tackling Alcohol Together: The Evidence Base for a UK Alcohol Policy. Free Association Books, London.

Raistrick, D., Heather, N., Godfrey, C., 2006. Review of the effectiveness of treatment for alcohol problems. National Treatment Agency for Substance Misuse. NHS.

Ray, G., Mertens, J., Weisner, C., 2009. Family members of people with alcohol or drug dependence: health and medical cost compared to family members of people with diabetes and asthma. Addiction 104, 203–214.

Rehm, J., Bauliunas, D., Borges, G., Graham, K., Irving, H., Kehoe, T., Parry, C., Patra, J., Popova, S., Poznyak, V., Roerecke, M., Room, R., Samokhvalov, A., Taylor, B., 2010. The relation between different dimensions of alcohol consumption and burden of disease: an overview. Addiction 105, 817–843.

Robertson, I., Heather, N., 1998. So you want to cut down your drinking? A self help guide to sensible drinking. Health Education Board Scotland, Edinburgh.

Rodger, J., 2008. Criminalising Social Policy: Anti-social Behaviour and Welfare in a De-civilised Society. Williams, Devon.

Rohsenow, D., Marlatt, A., 1981. The balanced placebo design: methodological considerations. Addict. Behav. 6, 107–122.

Roizen, R. Roizen's model. http://www.health.gov.au/internet/publications/publishing.nsf/Content/drugtreat-pubs-front6-oh-toc~drugtreat-pubs-front6-oh-11~drugtreat-pubs-front6-oh-11-3.

Room, R., Livingston, M., 2010. Who drinks how much less with which price policy? A rich feast for policy discussion. Addiction 105, 394–395.

Room, R., Rehm, J., 2011. Alcohol and non-communicable diseases – cancer heart disease and more. Addiction 106, 1–2.

Room, R., Babor, T., Rehm, J., 2005. Alcohol and public health. Lancet 365, 519–530.

Roozen, H., de Waart, R., van de Kroft, P., 2010. Community reinforcement and family training: an effective option to engage treatment resistant substance-abusing individuals in treatment. Addiction 105 (10), 1729–1738.

Ruidavets, J.-B., Ducimetière, P., Evans, A., Montaye, M., Haas, B., et al., 2010. Patterns of alcohol consumption and ischaemic heart disease in culturally divergent countries: the Prospective Epidemiological Study of Myocardial Infarction (PRIME). BMJ 341, c6077.

Rumpf, H., Bischof, G., Hapke, U., Meyer, C., John, U., 2000. Studies on natural recovery from alcohol dependence: sample selection bias by media solicitation? Addiction 95, 765–775.

Russell, M., 1994. New assessment tools for risk drinking during pregnancy: T-ACE, TWEAK and others. Alcohol Health Res. World 18, 55–61.

Salize, H., Jacke, C., Kief, S., Franz, M., Mann, K., 2013. Treating alcoholism reduces financial burden on caregivers and increases quality-adjusted life years. Addiction 108, 62–70.

SALSUS, 2008. National report. Smoking, drinking and drug use among 13 and 15 year olds in Scotland in 2008 Scottish Schools Adolescent Lifestyle and Substance Use Survey. NHS Scotland. www.drugmisuse.isdscotland.org/publications/abstracts/salsus.htm.

Saunders, W., Kershaw, P., 1979. Spontaneous remission from alcoholism – a community. Br. J. Addict. 74 (3), 251–265.

Schutze, M., Boeing, H., Pischon, T., Rehm, J., et al., 2011. Alcohol attributable burden of incidence of cancer in eight European countries based on results from prospective cohort study. BMJ 342, 1–10, d1584. http://dx.doi.org/10.1136/bmj.com.

Scottish Executive, 2002. Plan for action on alcohol abuse. Scottish Executive, Edinburgh.

Scottish Executive, 2003. Getting our priorities right: good practice guidance for working with children and families affected by substance misuse. Scottish Executive, Edinburgh.

Scottish Executive, 2004. Off-sales in the community: report of the working group on off-sales in the community. Scottish Executive, Edinburgh.

Scottish Executive, 2007. Licensing (Scotland) Act 2005: guidance for licensing boards and local authorities. Scottish Executive, Edinburgh.

Scottish Government, 2003. Mind the gaps – meeting the needs of people with co-occurring substance misuse and mental health problems. Report of the joint Working Group Scottish Advisory Committee on Drug Misuse (SACDM), Scottish Advisory Committee on Alcohol Misuse (SACAM). Scottish Executive, Edinburgh. www.scotland.gov.uk/Publications/2003/10/18358/28079.

Scottish Government, 2007. Plan for Action on Alcohol Problems. Scottish Government, Edinburgh. www.scotland.gov.uk/Publications/2007/02/19150222/0 (accessed 28 September 2011).

Scottish Government, 2008a. Changing Scotland's relationship with alcohol: a discussion paper on our strategic approach. Crown Copyright.

Scottish Government, 2008b. Equally well: report of the ministerial taskforce on health inequalities. Scottish Government, Edinburgh.

Scottish Government, 2009. A review of fixed penalty notices (FPN) for antisocial behaviour. Scottish Government. http://www.scotland.gov.uk/Publications/2009/11/24155814/4 (accessed 12 August 2011).

Scottish Government, 2010. National Guidance for Child Protection in Scotland 2010. Scottish Government.

Scottish Government, 2011. Alcohol brief interventions. http://www.scotland.gov.uk/About/Performance/scotPerforms/partnerstories/NHSScotlandperformance/alcoholbriefinterventions.

Scottish Intercollegiate Guidelines Network, 2003 Management of harmful drinking and alcohol dependence. Guideline 74. SIGN, Edinburgh.

Scottish Ministerial Advisory Committee on Alcohol Problems, 2011. Quality Alcohol Treatment SMACAP Scottish Government. Edinburgh.

Scottish Qualifications Authority. The Professional Development Award (PDA) in brief interventions for substance misuse. www.sqa.org.uk/sqa/48417.html (accessed 1 April 2014).

Shaw, S., Cartwright, J., Harwin, J., 1978. Responding to Drinking Problems. Croom Helm, London.

Shaw, J., Hunt, I.M., Flynn, S., Amos, T., Meehan, J., Robinson, J., Bickley, H., Parsons, R., McCann, K., Burns, J., Kapur, N., Appleby, L., 2006. The role of alcohol and drugs in homicides in England and Wales. Addiction 101, 1117–1124.

Slattery, J., Chick, J., Cochrane, M., Craig, J., Godfrey, C., Kohli, H., Macpherson, K., Parrot, S., Quinn, S., Single, A., Tochel, C., Watson, H., 2003. Prevention of relapse in alcohol dependence. Health Technology Assessment Report 3: Health Technology Board for Scotland, Glasgow.

Smit, E., Verdurman, J., Monshouwer, K., Smit, F., 2008. Family interventions and their effect on adolescent alcohol use in general populations; a meta-analysis of randomized controlled trials. Drug Alcohol Depend. 97 (3), 195–206.

Smith, L., Foxcroft, D., 2009. Drinking in the UK: an exploration of trends. Joseph Rowntree Foundation, York. www.jrf.org.uk.

Smith, S., Touquet, R., Wright, S., Das Gupta, N., 1996. Detection of alcohol-misusing patients in accident and emergency departments: the Paddington alcohol test (PAT). J. Accid. Emerg. Med. 13, 308–312.

Smith, P., Homish, G., Leonard, K., Cornelius, J., 2012. Women ending marriage to a problem drinking partner decrease their own risk for problem drinking. Addiction 107 (8), 1453–1461.

Sokol, R., Martier, S., Ager, J., 1989. The T-ACE questions: practical prenatal detection of risk-drinking. Am. J. Obstet. Gynecol. 160, 863–870.

Sondhi, A., Turner, C., 2011. The influence of family and friends on young peoples' drinking. Joseph Rowntree Foundation.www.jrf.org.uk.

References

Stockwell, T., Gruenewald, P., 2004. Controls on the physical availability of alcohol. In: Heather, N., Stockwell, T. (Eds.), The Essential Handbook of Treatment and Prevention of Alcohol Problems. Wiley & Sons, England.

Stockwell, T., Zhao, J., Macdonald, S., Pakula, B., Gruenwald, P., Holder, H., 2009. Changes in per capita alcohol sales during the partial privatization of British Columbia's retail alcohol monopoly 2003–2008: a multi level local area analysis. Addiction 104, 1827–1836.

Tiffany, S., 1990. A cognitive model of drug urges and drug-use behavior: role of automatic and nonautomatic processes. Psychol. Rev. 97, 147–168.

Tobutt, C. (Ed.), 2011. Alcohol at work: managing alcohol problems and issues in the workplace, Gower.

Trade Union Congress. http://www.tuc.org.uk/workplace/drugsandalcohol.cfm (accessed 1 April 2014).

TWEAK Test. http://alcoholism.about.com/od/tests/a/tweak.htm (accessed 1 April 2014).

UKATT Research Team, 2008. UK Alcohol Treatment Trial: client treatment matching effects. Addiction 103, 228–238.

Vaillant, G., 1983. The Natural History of Alcoholism. Harvard University Press, Cambridge.

Vaillant, G., 2003. A 60-year follow-up of alcoholic men. Addiction 98, 1043–1051.

Vaillant, G., Milofsky, E., 1982. Natural history of male alcoholism. IV. Paths to recovery. Arch. Gen. Psychiatry 39 (2), 127–133.

Valentine, G., Jayne, M., et al., 2010. Family life and alcohol consumption: a study of transmission of drinking practices. Joseph Rowntree Foundation, York.

Wagenaar, A., 1993. Minimum drinking age and alcohol availability to youth: issues and research needs. In: Hilton, M., Bloss, G. (Eds.), Economics and the Prevention of Alcohol-Related Problems. NIAAA, Bethesda.

Wagenaar, A.C., Salois, M.J., Komro, K., 2009. Effects of beverage alcohol price and tax levels on drinking: a meta analysis of 1003 estimates from 112 studies. Addiction 104, 179–190.

Wales, A., Gillan, E., 2009. Untold damage: children's accounts of living with harmful parental drinking. SHAAP/ ChildLine, Edinburgh.

Watson, H., Godfrey, C., et al., 2009. Reducing alcohol-related harm in the workplace: a feasibility study of screening and brief intervention for hazardous drinkers. Alcohol Research UK, London. http://alcoholresearchuk.org/2009/ 02/10/reducing-alcohol-related-harm-in-the-workplace-a-feasibility-study-of-screening-and-brief-interventions-for-hazardous-drinkers (accessed 1 August 2013).

Watson, H., Munro, A., Wilson, M., Kerr, S., Godwin, J., 2011. The involvement of nurses and midwives in screening and brief interventions for hazardous and harmful use of alcohol and other psychoactive substances. World Health Organisation.

Weaver, T., Madden, P., Charles, V., Stimson, G., et al., 2003. Comorbidity of substance misuse and mental illness in community mental health and substance misuse services. Br. J. Psychiatry 183, 3003–3313.

White, W., 2007. Addiction recovery: its definition and conceptual boundaries. J. Subst. Abuse Treat. 33 (3), 229–241.

Williams, D., Lowdown on the high street. Observer Food Monthly. No 119. Observer. 2011, London.

World Health Organisation, 1992. International Classification of Diseases, Tenth Revision (ICD-10). WHO. http:// www.who.int/classifications/icd/en/bluebook.pdf.

World Health Organisation, 1993. International Statistical Classification of Disease and Health-Related Problems. ICD-10. WHO, Geneva.

World Health Organisation, 1994. Lexicon of Alcohol and Drug Terms. WHO, Geneva.

World Health Organisation Europe, 2009. Handbook for action to reduce alcohol related harm. Geneva. www.euro. who.int/__data/assets/pdf_file/0012/43320/E92820.pdf (accessed 16 April 2014).

World Health Organisation Europe, 2010. European status report on alcohol and health. WHO.

Young, R., Sweeting, H., West, P., 2007. A longitudinal study of alcohol use and antisocial behaviour in young people. Alcohol Alcohol. 43 (2), 204–214. www.ncbi.nlm.nih.gov/pmc/articles/PMC2367698.

Index

Note: Page numbers followed by *b* indicate boxes and *t* indicate tables.

Index